YOU ARE WHAT YOU ATE

An Rx for the resistant diseases of the 21st century

Sherry A. Rogers, M.D.
F.A.C.A.I., F.A.A.E.M., F.A.A.F.P.

Prestige Publishing
P.O. Box 3068, 3502 Brewerton Road, Syracuse, NY 13220
1-800-846-6687 • 315-455-7862 • Fax 315-454-8119
http://www.prestigepublishing.com

Printing History:
    First Edition:
        1st Printing - April, 1988
        2nd Printing - July, 1989
    Second Edition:
        1st Printing - January, 1990
    Third Edition:
        1st Printing – September, 1997
        2nd Printing – January, 2000

Library of Congress Catalog Card Number: 95-068457

ISBN 0-9618821-8-2

For information address to:
    Prestige Publishing
    P.O. Box 3068
    Syracuse, NY 13220

    1-800-846-6687, 315-455-7862, Fax 315-454-8119
    http://www.prestigepublishing.com

Printed in the United States

TABLE OF CONTENTS

DEDICATION
DISCLAIMER
FOREWORD
PREFACE TO 2ND EDITION

Sherry A. Rogers, M.D., F.A.C.A.I., F.A.B.E.M., F.A.B.F.P.
Northeast Center for Environmental Medicine
2800 West Genesee Street
Syracuse, NY 13219

Mail correspondence to:
P.O. Box 2716
Syracuse, NY 13220

1997

DEDICATION

To Rob, my most precious gift from God, who nearly starved to death while discovering that he hates macrobiotic food. Eighteen years ago when we were bride and groom, little did I suspect that a love so strong could grow even more wonderful through the years. Nor did I ever dream that in addition to this indescribable blessing, my groom would continually nourish and groom me into all that I was capable of being.

And to our staff, in particular Barbara Mulvana, Shirley Gallinger, Carol Fenton, and Frank Mulvana, who over many years, through computer crashes and hectic days have worked diligently to help patients learn and grow along with us in our quest for health.

DISCLAIMER

This work is a guide for people who are working in concert with a certified health professional. It is in no way meant to be a prescription for anyone attempting to heal themselves without medical monitoring and guidance.

FOREWORD

WHAT OTHER PHYSICIANS AND BIOCHEMISTS HAVE TO SAY ABOUT THIS BOOK

In this book, Dr. Rogers discusses many aspects of what some doctors now recognize as "environmental illness", called "E.I." for short. Many strictly orthodox medical practitioners are skeptical of the existence of E.I.; indeed a few are downright antagonistic toward this classification of illness.

As a biochemist, I speak from a rather unique vantage point. For ten years I have operated a consulting organization for medical practices nationwide. We have had the opportunity to do detailed studies of individuals who present particularly severe intolerances to foods, environmental chemicals, inhalant allergens and other substances. My colleagues and I have extensive files of very orthodox, very authoritative clinical laboratory results on measurements such as: enzyme activities in blood cells, plasma and urine levels of amino acids and fatty acids, vitamin and mineral levels in different tissues and body fluids, immune profiles, standard blood chemistry profiles, results of cultures of foreign flora, gastrointestinal work-ups, blood screens for foreign chemicals (pesticides, herbicides, fungicides, petroleum solvents), etc. WE have studied and consulted on over 2300 individuals who have had such extensive biochemical work-ups. Some of these work-ups are for various degenerative diseases, some are for genetic illnesses, some are for behavioral or developmental disabilities, and many are for people who can be classed as presenting E.I. In summary, we have hard laboratory data, comparisons with normal levels, documented symptoms observed and all reported by many doctors throughout the world (over 150). Therefore, we have an informed opinion.

In almost all cases of E.I., we have identified an underlying deficit or dysfunction in essential nutrients, metabolism, or immune response. I believe that, for the few where we haven't found the underlying problem, the fault lies in the incompleteness of available laboratory tests. Provocation and perpetuation of E.I. requires two conditions:

1. existence of a nutritional deficit or metabolic fault,

2. exposure to or contamination by a substance (perhaps just a single food) whose metabolism or detoxication does not proceed properly because of item (1).

This is to be distinguished from an acute toxic exposure where toxicity would result regardless of the individual's metabolism. We have to recognize the difference between acute toxicity and sub-acute or chronic conditions where the body's detoxication processes are impaired such that "chemical sensitivities", "food allergies", "universal reactivity" become genuine conditions. If we just observe our acquaintances, we begin to see the problem. One individual may have the ability to drive through traffic, work in a steel plant in the midst of pollution, and return home via the neighborhood bar, while another individual may develop a debilitating headache just from auto exhaust on the commute to his place of work. Individual tolerances vary tremendously as do individual metabolisms. In pristine environments, this individuality should be apparent to the profession, nutritionists, and to people at large.

The two factors initiating E.I. that are stated above enable two treatment modalities to be valid and effective. One modality, the oldest in environmental medicine or clinical ecology, is the identification of the provoking substances and removal of those substances from the individual's environment. Alternatively, the individual may remove himself from the site of the provoking substance. This modality addresses item (2) above. Fasting, careful washing of food, cleaning the home, ridding the home of fungal growths and volatile household chemicals are examples. The second modality is nutritional, metabolic or immunologic. Using laboratory or in office tests, the doctor treats the individual's nutritional, metabolic or immunologic faults. This second modality increases tolerance and may provide a more lasting benefit. It is as important as the first modality because we can't hide forever from our environment.

In this book, Dr. Rogers discusses macrobiotic diets. Macrobiotic diets avoid highly refined carbohydrates (sugars), most fats, food additives, and most xenobiotic contaminants. (What's xenobiotic? Read this book!) Actually, a macrobiotic diet can be a modality that addresses item (2) above – such a diet can remove provoking substances. I have studied the nutritional and metabolic status of individuals who have been on macrobiotic diets for months, some for years. I have seen some individuals with recurrent malignancies stop the recurrence while on such a diet. For others, unfortunately, the strategy didn't work. Also, I observed the development of nutritional deficits, such as iron deficiency and anemia for individuals on macrobiotic diets. So, a word of warning. When on a restricted diet, have your doctor do a nutritional work-up form time to time. Many clinical laboratories now offer: quantitative blood vitamin levels, whole blood or blood cell mineral levels, and blood or urine amino acid profiles. These tests are wise investments, and I endorse them.

I urge you to purchase and read this book because it may tell you what is wrong with you or what is going to go wrong with you. If so, then the book also shows you how to alleviate the situation through better environmental awareness and perhaps through dietary changes. Most importantly, it should help you communicate with health professionals, doctors and nutritionists about your environmental illness.

Jon Pangborn, Ph.D., F.A.I.C.
President, BIONOSTICS, INC.
Lisle, IL 60532

Dr. Rogers is again leading the way with her own personal experimentation. The adaptation of the rotary diversified diet with the macrobiotic program should be an advance for those people who don't have total success with either along. She has personally found that this modification was the next step in her search for optimum health.

I whole heartedly agree with her modification and hope that this will help others.

William J Rea, M.D., F.A.C.S., F.A.A.E.M., F.A.C.A.I.
Founder, Environmental Health Center, Dallas,
Thoracic and Cardiovascular Surgeon,
First World Professorial Chair in Environmental Medicine
Robens Institute, University of Surrey, England

Sherry Rogers' primary goal is to make people consciously aware of the options and choices from which they can choose a more healthy lifestyle. She presents her ideas with elegant simplicity. This really indicates how clearly she herself has considered the issues. To educate or to medicate? As so often is the case, choosing the more difficult path involves elevating the individual to a higher state of understanding, to a cleaner lifestyle, and to a less indulgent handling of life's dilemmas. There are endless details to be considered by the environmentally ill patient or the individual who consciously chooses a less chemically contaminate lifestyle. Each of these details in themselves is not so important. However, the awareness that Sherry directs toward these details is the critical issue. Her simple and elegant presentation is inspiring and does the one thing that a great work must do. It inspires us to spiral upward and try to bring more awareness to every detail of our everyday lives. Thanks so much for this loving work.

Stephen A. Levine, Ph.D.
President, Nutricology Inc.
San Leandro, CA 94577
Author, ANTIOXIDANT ADAPTATION

Sherry A. Rogers, M.D. has been a pioneer in the field of E.I. combining shrewd observation with an inquiring scientific mind, she has advanced our understanding of E.I. and has provided objective data for the skeptics. As one of the most accomplished physicians in the field, Dr. Rogers has attracted some of the sicker and more complicated patients to her practice.

In this book, Dr. Rogers discusses the possibility that macrobiotics may be the answer for some patients who have not found adequate relief from their chronic problems. Macrobiotics is difficult to explain from a Western scientific viewpoint, but any treatment that helps a substantial percentage of the most difficult-to-treat patients is worthy of additional investigation.

YOU ARE WHAT YOU ATE attempts to incorporate the macrobiotic approach into the Western medical model. Some devotees of the former might be unhappy with Dr. Rogers' rejection of some aspects of the macrobiotic philosophy. However, she correctly points out that an ancient discipline may require modification in this nutrient-depleted, chemically overloaded age. In this book, Dr. Rogers has made a creditable attempt to merge the best of environmental medicine and macrobiotics, two extremely complex and sometimes contradictory disciplines.

Alan R. Gaby, M.D.
Author, VITAMIN B6, THE NATURAL HEALER
Coauthor, NUTRITIONAL THERAPY IN MEDICAL PRACTICE
Editor, TOWNSEND LETTER FOR DOCTORS
Pikesville, MD 21208

PREFACE TO THE 2ND EDITION

Much has changed since the first edition of YOU ARE WHAT YOU ATE in 1988. At that point in time, it was written with much trepidation. For thinking that food had anything to do with wellness was next to quackery. To suggest that food, furthermore, had anything to do with healing such impossible conditions as chemical sensitivity or cancers, was unspeakable.

Nevertheless in 1988, we dared write YOU ARE WHAT YOU ATE because we knew that in spite of all of the macrobiotic books, no physician had looked at macrobiotics as a relative newcomer with a sense of humor and much skepticism. Thus it turned out to be the first book on macrobiotics written by a medical doctor or dissect macrobiotics from both sides, addressing the pros and the cons with a sense of humor, and with the special patient with allergies, chemical sensitivity, E.I., and Candida problems in mind.

Since that edition in 1988, much has happened in the last 7 years. First we wrote TIRED OR TOXIC? Which has over 33 biochemical mechanisms of why macrobiotics is able to heal the impossible. And in fact, since recommending macrobiotics to hundreds of patients with E.I. (environmental illness), we have watched them, as well as ourselves, overcome this 21st century disease. In fact, many people from around the world have written in thanking us for writing it, because they also went on the macrobiotic diet and cleared their symptoms. We also have had the privilege of witnessing people who have reversed impossible cancers. Many of them have been kind enough to send their stories, their x-ray reports, their doctors' reports, and all the medical substantiation.

For example, Melissa from New England is a lovely young lady who developed an inoperable brain tumor in her 30's. She was given less than 6 months to live and had consulted numerous specialists. When she cleared her tumor with the macrobiotic diet and went back to her doctor showing him the negative brain scans, he was incredulous and then decided that he and all of the other consultants, and the x-rays, and the vision tests showing quadrant blindness must have been in error. So you can understand that acceptance of macrobiotics still has been and continues to be very difficult for the average medical professional.

In spite of this resistance, we rolled along having more and more people go on the macrobiotic diet. Then it became very apparent to us that we had to have a book that would take people beyond YOU ARE WHAT YOU ATE and describe the strict healing phase diet in explicit detail. So I went to the top, to the foremost macrobiotic specialist in the world, Mr. Michio Kushi. I explained worriedly that if something happened to him, a great deal of wonderful knowledge would be lost. Someone should write down what his explicit consultation is that may people used who have successfully cleared their cancers. For many have totally healed and even gone on to write their autobiographies.

One very convincing autobiography was that of Elaine Nussbaum. After you have read her story, RECOVERY, no physicians with a clear conscience could help but recommend macrobiotics to their patients. In her 30's, she developed cancer of the ovaries and had a hysterectomy, but the cancer spread to the lungs and liver. She had chemotherapy and radiation and still the cancer spread to the back bones which collapsed. Within 2 years she was bedridden, bald, 78 pounds, racked with pain, unable to walk, and the cancer was still spreading. She also had pneumonia and at this point her doctors said that they didn't even dare give her an antibiotic for her pneumonia, because she was so frail and only had a few weeks to live and the antibiotic might kill her prematurely. At this point, she went on the macrobiotic diet. That was 9 years ago. I was lecturing with her last summer as usual at the Kushi Summer Conference, and when I met up with her she had just come in from jogging. She is totally well.

Anyway, Mr. Kushi graciously invited me to come to Boston as much as I needed. And so I flew to Boston every month for 6 months writing down everything he advised people who came from literally all parts of the globe. When I would go home I would study the notes voraciously, and when by the last trip I could write what he was going to tell them to eat 2 minutes before it came out of his mouth, and for 3 days straight, I knew I had the program. Hence, the birth of THE CURE IS IN THE KITCHEN.

We thought we were done writing macrobiotic books at that time, but another problem arose. We realized that we had to figure out what to feed the rest of the family who turned up their noses at macrobiotics and said "Eek! I'm not going to eat that stuff." Our gifted nurse, Shirley Gallinger, wrote MACRO MELLOW, which shows people how to disguise the macro foods as delicious "normal looking" foods that the rest of the family would eat. In this way, it unloads the cook tremendously (who oftentimes is the patient as well). The cook doesn't have to spend time cooking double meals. She can dress up macrobiotics for the rest of the family and keep out a little of the plain unadulterated portions for the person on the strict healing phase. Also, MACRO MELLOW is great for people who realize that they are not quite ready to do the macrobiotic diet and so it helps them ease into more healthful cooking slowly. Mrs. Gallinger, the author of MACRO MELLOW, gives not only recipes and menus, but kitchen organizational, shopping and garden hints. Hence, we now had a 3 part macro almanac: the primer (YOU ARE WHAT YOU ATE), the complete strict healing phase (THE CURE IS IN THE KITCHEN), and the directions to make it acceptable to the rest of the family (MACRO MELLOW).

She herself is a perfect example of what macrobiotics can do. She has healed all of the medical problems that she has had in the past and as well is an active member on the ski patrol, and motorcycled on her vacations from Syracuse to Colorado and from Syracuse to Nova Scotia. No easy trick for a woman in her mid 60's. Meanwhile, the world is learning about the power of macrobiotics.

In LANCET (a very prestigious British medical journal) in 1990, Dr. Dean Ornish published how they had reversed coronary artery disease in people for whom all else had failed. They had had by-pass surgery, they were on cholesterol lowering drugs, and they were still clotting off new vessels. They were slated to be dead within 5 years from a second coronary. Instead a group of them elected to go on the macrobiotic diet and within 1 year they had reversed the arteriosclerosis as proven on PET scans.

Likewise, Carter and his colleagues published in the 1993 JOURNAL OF THE AMERICAN COLLEGE OF NUTRITION (12:13, 205), a wonderful article showing that you can more than triple your survival from cancers by using the macrobiotic diet. For example, they showed that if you do everything that medicine has to offer for cancer of the prostate including surgery, chemo-therapy, radiation, and hormones, that the median survival is only 6 years. However, if you do the macrobiotic diet, median survival is 19 years. And the hooker was, in order to qualify for the macrobiotic group, you only had to be on the diet a minimum of 3 months. So many of these 3 monthers brought the 19 year average down, because as many of you know, there are many of these people still alive who had cleared their prostatic cancers through the macrobiotic diet.

Medicine is slowly catching on and now they are actually taking foods apart and analyzing them for their constituents that are responsible for changing the cancer cells, namely phyto-chemicals. One of the phyto-chemicals for example, is called sulforaphane. The Brassica family (broccoli, kohlrabi, mustard greens, cauliflower, Brussels sprouts, turnips, kale, collards, etc.) is rich in this phyto chemical it turns out, and this phyto-chemical not only is able to prevent cancers, but it also can reverse them. But unfortunately, rather than recommending more of these foods and the macrobiotic diet, medicine is trying to figure out how to make synthetic sulforaphane that can be put into a pill form and then marketed as an expensive drug treatment for cancers.

We also discovered some other interesting things since the first edition of this book and that is that some people are definitely not macrobiotic material. So don't force your spouse or other people into it if they feel that they need meat. You can learn all about these carnivores and how they have cleared cancers in WELLNESS AGAINST ALL ODDS. And if you have trouble with your insurance company helping you for your consultations, you should read and use THE SCIENTIFIC BASIS FOR SELECTED ENVIRONMENTAL MEDICINE TECHNIQUES.

CHEMICAL SENSITIVITY is an inexpensive, referenced booklet to teach physicians and lay alike about one of the unknown reasons that hold people back from healing. And regardless of your diagnostic label, our 9th book, DEPRESSION CURED AT LAST!, contains new information about healing, above and beyond all the others.

So what's next? I don't know where it is going to end, because there are so many fresh ideas, new facts, and research data that come out everyday that I don't know how to get the information out to people fast enough. So as well as the 9 books, we have a monthly subscription newsletter (which is also referenced for physicians) called TOTAL HEALTH IN TODAY'S WORLD so that people can continually grow and keep abreast of new findings.

When all has been said and done, one thing is for sure, and that is that eating close to nature is definitely a key to wellness. Medicine is slowly catching up and discovering the scientific explanation and proof for why and how all of this works. Yet, they are still ignoring it in place of expensive drugs and surgery, which keep the medical industry fluid. But for perennially tired people or people who are not well, and definitely for people who do not have enough money for medical care, with all I know from a quarter of a century medical practice and research, I would recommend starting with a macrobiotic diet. For even if you find out that it is not for you, it is an excellent start from which you can always switch to the programs in WELLNESS AGAINST ALL ODDS. And a new cancer book with even more exciting data, above and beyond the rest, is due in 1998.

Fortunately for the majority of people, simply changing to a macrobiotic diet has been a major change to wellness. And it is not a life sentence. For after you have become well, you can back off and have a much more lenient diet and have periodic splurges of all of your old favorites. So let's get started and learn about this wonderful God-given program.

Sherry A. Rogers, M.D.
1997

CHAPTER I
INTRODUCTION
WHO CARRIES THE BALL?

Do you want to get well?

Do you want to awaken after five hours of sleep playful,
laughing and enthusiastic to tackle the day?

Do you want to reach new levels of wellness,
physically and mentally?

Then you have chosen "educate".
For in the world of medicine there are only two choices:

TO MEDICATE OR EDUCATE

If you prefer to medicate, you choose conventional medicine
where symptoms are given an accepted term or name
(diagnosis). Then blood tests and x-rays are done to confirm
that the accepted term has been correctly applied to this
conglomeration of symptoms. After that, it is merely a matter
of trial and error to determine which drug will relieve all the
symptoms. If success is not imminent, surgery is considered.
Next case.

For example: Mr. Jones complains of a headache.

Through the diagnostic process he has a chemical
profile and CAT scan.

He receives a magic label: "Mr. Jones, you have
migraines".

1

To medicate

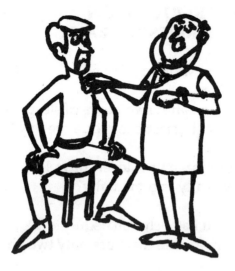

or

educate——

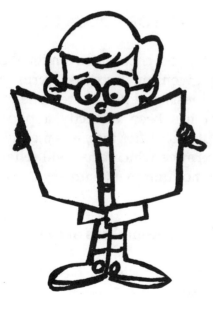

That is the question.

He gets his treatment: a prescription for pain pills and migraine pills.

Mr. Jones goes home to watch T.V. and drinks beer and eats chocolate and has a migraine.

What's wrong? Mr. Jones has chosen a doctor who does not search for a cause of symptoms. He merely medicates. He thinks a headache is a codeine deficiency. Furthermore, he has given the unspoken message to Mr. Jones: eat, drink, and breathe whatever you want. I have a pill for everything.

On the other hand, if Mr. Jones wants to take an active part in his health and find the causes for his symptoms and get rid of them without medication, this requires work. He must be educated. This takes time and insurance companies don't pay for time spent in educating patients. Also, Mr. Jones will have to seek out a physician trained in finding causes and interested in educating the patient. And he has to learn to listen to his body----not just when it belts him between the eyes, but when it whispers in his ear. And Mr. Jones will have to modify his lifestyle. He will have to read that boring book, **THE E.I. SYNDROME, REVISED.** But he has a choice: To medicate or educate.

And the choice extends far beyond the present illness. It extends to his day to day well-being and his overall life span. For the decision he makes today will have an effect on all his other symptoms and even his future decision-making process itself.

So the very first thing Mr. Jones has to decide is to whom will he give responsibility for his health? His doctor or himself? Who is going to carry the ball?

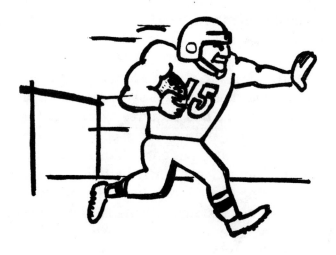

And who is going to carry the ball for your health?

Your doctor is your coach or consultant. You are the player who decides whether the game is won. Don't make the coach carry the ball. No one ever won that way.

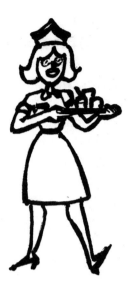

Every medicine
has its side
effects and
drawbacks and
merely masks
symptoms.

Many people take
extra drugs to
cover the side
effects of their
primary drugs.

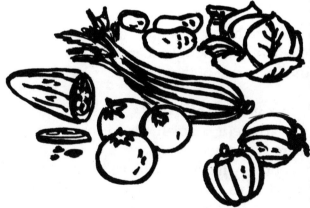

Every medicine
puts an extra
stress on the
body's
detoxification
system.

Why not have your
food be your
medicine
while first
strengthening your
detox system with
appropriate
nutrients?

CHAPTER II
E.I. IN A NUTSHELL

E.I., or environmental illness, can masquerade as many common medical symptoms and diseases: migraines, chronic exhaustion, recurrent infection, chronic post nasal drip, asthma, bronchitis, irritable bowel, colitis, spastic colon, chronic cystitis, traumatic arthritis, vasculitis, sarcoid, lupus, eczema, psoriasis, Sjogren's syndrome, depression, spaciness, inability to concentrate, hyperactivity, violent mood swings, urethritis, prostatitis, TMJ (temporomandibular joint), chronic EBV (Epstein Barr Virus), rheumatoid arthritis, degenerative arthritis, neuritis, endometriosis, dizziness, chronic Candida, chemical hypersensitivity, infertility, poor memory, panic attacks, weakness and many undiagnosable maladies. For more information, consult our 650 page book, **THE E.I. SYNDROME, REVISED** (Prestige Publishing, Box 3068, 1-800-846-6687, 3502 Brewerton Rd, Syracuse, NY 13220, $17.95 plus $4.00 S & H).

The ecologic approach to health has brought health answers and wellness to people who never thought they could be free of symptoms again. And I was one of these people.

However, in a small percentage of people, the ecologic approach is not enough. There is a small group for whom nothing has helped. There is another much larger group who are 50 to 95% improved, but they have not achieved that 100% that they know they could have. We've discovered further alternatives that are available for those who know that clean food and water, rotation diets, good environmental controls for pollens, dusts, molds land chemicals, correction of nutritional deficiencies, reduction of stress and hypo-sensitizing injections are not quite enough.

6

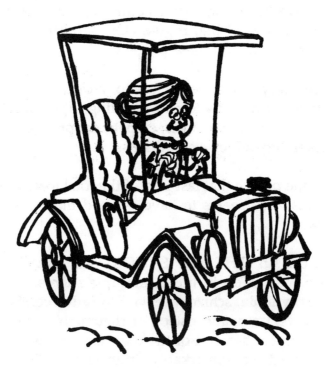

Age has nothing to do with fatigue and exhaustion. That is one of medicine's many cop-outs or myths.

For these people, their bodies are still not unloaded enough, in spite of having worked through the total load, to allow them to heal. Some of them are so sensitive, they cannot even come out of their homes: they react to every chemical that abounds in the world outside of their bedrooms or an environmental unit. With the thousands of cases that have been observed during the practice of environmental medicine, we have seen one astounding fact; **the body can heal just about anything, if given the opportunity**. So what has arrested healing for these people?

For some, they have neglected to reduce their chemical environment sufficiently to allow healing. They still live with gas appliances or wood stoves, carpets, eat processed foods or work under very adverse conditions.

But for some people that last part of the total load seems to be far too illusive, it seems to have escaped their grasp; that is until now.

You'll recall in **THE E.I. SYNDROME, REVISED** how diagnoses of sarcoidosis, lupus, multiple sclerosis, intractable cardiac arrhythmia, schizophrenia, ulcerative colitis, arthritis (degenerative, traumatic, osteo-, or rheumatoid arthritis), and a multitude of other end-of-the-road conditions were either totally cleared or remarkably improved. Those people lovingly taught me that I should never stop looking for solutions, regardless of how narrowly I viewed a prognosis.

When we closely evaluate why some people are not better, it's obvious: they are just plain not sick enough to do all that is necessary. And that's all right. They have been educated and have chosen their paths. We all have a certain time when we choose to make time to coordinate a health program. The missing part of the total load boat varies from person to person. But here's a quick checklist to be sure you have done all you can up to this point to heal your environmental illness or E.I. And bear in mind E.I. really encompasses every chronic symptom of unwellness that does not yet merit a name by the current medical system. In the following total load synopsis, obviously not everyone needs everything that is listed. But you should persist until you are free of symptoms. And if symptoms still persist, then the remainder of this book is for you.

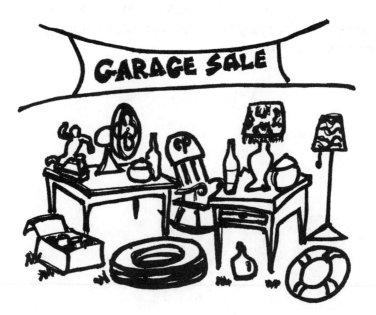

Get rid of as much junk as possible from your home, especially in the bedroom oasis. Why have things outgassing and collecting dust that you will never use?

E.I. CHECKLIST

Is your inhalant load covered?

_____ 1. Have you exposed mold plates in the bedroom and other places you most commonly frequent? If the mold is high, have you recultured until the plates show your environmental controls are good? Anyone can send for petri dishes or mold plates to expose in the home. Directions are included plus a return mailer. A list of the types and numbers of molds identified by a Ph.D. mycologist will be mailed to you as soon as the last mold has stopped growing. This is usually within 2-7 weeks. Petri dishes or mold plates, as they are called, are available from Mold Survey Service, PO Box 2716, Syracuse, NY 13220.

_____ 2. Is there an air cleaner in the bedroom, regularly serviced?

_____ 3. Is the carpet out of the bedroom?

_____ 4. Is there an air conditioner in the bedroom?

_____ 5. Has there been removal of all objects except the bed if you are very sensitive (especially bureaus and closet contents)?

_____ 6. Has there been cutting of nearby trees, installing gutters, trenches, and dry wells about the house to reduce dampness; corrections of leaks, removal of old wallpaper, bathroom tiles, and other hidden sources of mold?

____ 7. Test titrated inhalants (pollens, dust, molds, mites) and receive injections twice weekly until symptoms are clear. Return to twice weekly interval if symptoms recur.

____ 8. Break down mixes (trees, grasses, molds) and test to individual components of mixes that are especially allergenic.

____ 9. Test new molds.

____10. Retest phenol and glycerin if injections cause a problem.

____11. Do you have cotton mattress covers and bedding, regularly washed? Did you evaluate foil on the covered mattress?

____12. Is there regular wet dusting to remove and not merely redistribute the dust?

____13. Did you remove allergenic animals?

Has food allergy been ruled out?
____ 1. Use glass bottled spring water for a one month trial.

____ 2. Did you evaluate the rare food, rotated diet for one month?

____ 3. If there was no difference, a different rare food diet, not necessarily rotated of extremely rare foods and as organic as possible should be evaluated on the chance that your initial one contained hidden food allergies.

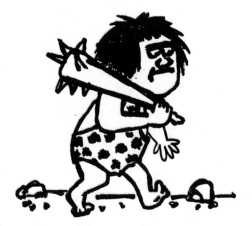

The caveman diet or rare food diet is a must for anyone who doesn't feel wonderful. Hidden food allergies are extremely common.

_____ 4. Have you fasted five days?

_____ 5. Did you evaluate food testing and daily injections for a least 6 months?

_____ 6. Did you look for intestinal hyperpermeability, the leading cause and perpetuator of food allergies? (see **WELLNESS AGAINST ALL ODDS**)

Is Candida a problem?

_____ 1. Did you do a ferment-free (bread, cheese, alcohol, vinegar, catsup, mayonnaise, salad dressing, packaged foods) and sugar-free (nothing with corn syrup, maple syrup, cane sugar, dextrose, maltose, malt, honey) diet for two months?

_____ 2. With a known reputable source of acidophilus such as Vital Dophilus used for 6 months?

_____ 3. Did you evaluate a trial of Nystatin with all of the above for 2 months?

_____ 4. And the addition of 2-4 week trial of ketoconazole (Nizoral) or other systemic anti-fungal?

Is there a hidden nutritional deficiency?

_____ 1. Have all the latest vitamin and mineral assays been drawn? There are new tests available every few months, that we didn't have before.

_____ 2. Have special tests for amino acids and essential fatty acids been drawn?

14

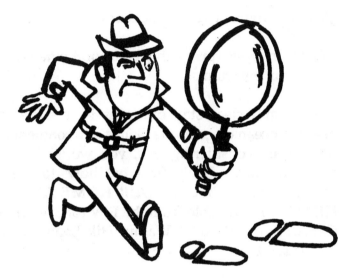

In your search for wellness, follow methodically the ecologic checklist for clues of areas you have missed. Reread THE E.I. SYNDROME, REVISED.

_____ 3. Correct deficiencies then reassess the balance.

_____ 4. Make a special appointment to assess biochemical nutritional status and diet quality.

_____ 5. Check for unsuspected glandular or endocrine problems like DHEA deficiency or hypothyroidism or hypoglycemia or testosterone deficiency.

The toughest problem: The chemical environment.

_____ 1. Create an oasis (preferably bedroom) where you can clear your symptoms.

_____ 2. If you can't clear, stay outdoors in a safe area like near the ocean or go to the Dallas environmental unit. (If you are considering this, you would be wise to read Dr. Rea's book first on how to build an ecologically safe house. **YOUR HOME AND YOUR HEALTH** is available from the Environmental Health Center, Suite 200, 8345 Walnut Hill Lane, Dallas, TX 75231, $20.)

_____ 3. Go on oxygen temporarily.

_____ 4. Only after you are clear can you reenter environments to identify the culprits. Some of the worst triggers are urea foam formaldehyde insulated buildings, tight buildings, traffic and industrial exhausts, gas heating systems and appliances, glues and adhesives (carpet, tiles, cupboards, furnishings), gasoline (benzene) and oils (pumps, furnaces, machines), plastics and synthetic materials (xylene, formaldehyde, toluene, acrylics, vinyls, benzene,

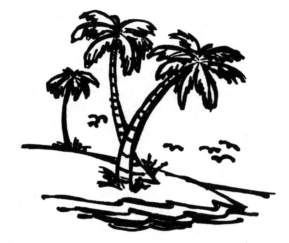

You need a home oasis, usually the bedroom. If you can't awaken feeling great, where are you going the rest of the day?

phenol), cleaning solutions and air-fresheners (xylene, benzene, trichloroethylene, phenol), pesticides, and municipal water (chlorine, chloroform).

_____ 5. Chemical-free personal grooming is mandatory: no scented cosmetics, deodorants, mousses, shampoos, soaps, lotions, sprays, astringents, conditioners, new fabrics, polyester or acrylic, dry cleaned items, detergents, fabric softeners or cigarette smoke.

_____ 6. Have plenty of fans and vents in the home and office: fresh (and filtered if in contaminated area) incoming air, adequate enough to displace outgassed chemicals.

_____ 7. Allow 1/2-2 years in a chemically clean environment (on a sound ecologic program with periodic monitoring) for healing to occur. It takes time. Only drugs give responses overnight.

_____ 8. Remove yourself from contaminants as soon as possible, shower, cleanse the bowel, take antioxidants and recover as quickly as possible.

_____ 9. Do you need to test chemicals? Do you need a test to see if you are overloaded and which part of your detox path is damaged?

_____10. Do you need a detoxification program?

_____11. Have you reread THE E.I. SYNDROME, REVISED?, TIRED OR TOXIC?, WELLNESS AGAINST ALL ODDS? Do you subscribe to the monthly newsletter? Do you keep abreast of new findings?

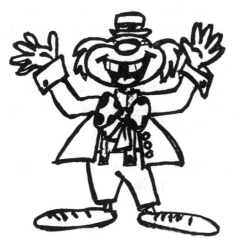

A sense of humor has long been known as a stimulant to the immune system. If you don't have a healthy one, get some professional counseling to see what holds you back.

Is your brain in a healing mode?

_____ 1. Do you need to be ill? Are you more comfortable being ill than well? If so, you need a professional counselor.

_____ 2. Do you practice positive imagery and not just wishful thinking?

_____ 3. Have you reduced your personal stress to show your body that you respect and love it? Are you making a commitment to lifestyle changes and wellness?

_____ 4. Have you changed your schedule to purposely make time for exercise, meditation and healing? Or are you still clinging to the excuse that you don't have time to make yourself well?

_____ 5. Do you frequently involve yourself with "up", happy, positive people?

_____ 6. Do you make sure you sing and laugh several times a day?

_____ 7. Do you set realistic goals and periodically assess your progress?

_____ 8. Do you feel optimistic and believe you are worth the effort, and that you will get well?

_____ 9. Do you have a firm spirituality that keeps maturing?

Have you ruled out special problems? For example:

____ 1. The need to have another thorough medical exam?

____ 2. Test hormones or neurotransmitters

____ 3. Test ionization and electromagnetic field effects.

____ 4. A non-supportive spouse

____ 5. Consider the new findings that do not yet exist in print. For this you should devour all the other books then schedule a time to brainstorm about the remaining possibilities.

Note: The above areas (2, 3, 5) are so new your only recourse will be to see the doctor for an explanation of these. They are not written up yet.

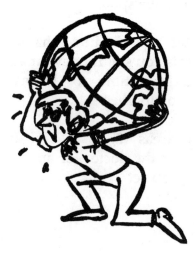

Everyone has problems. But some people don't choose to lessen their burdens in order to allow healing to proceed. Try to level with yourself or get professional help.

HEALING CANCERS

In searching for a clue to see why a small sector of people afflicted with environmental illness could not attain total recovery, I started looking at cancer patients. I discovered that there were people who had healed cancers that were termed incurable. For example, Dr. Anthony Satilaro, (author of **RECALLED BY LIFE**, Avon Books, a division of Hearst Corporation, 1970 Broadway, New York, NY 10019, 1984) was a physician in his mid forties who had cancer of the prostate which metastasized to the skull. He was given a maximum of three to six months to live by all of his colleagues who were specialists in various aspects of his treatment. As a director of a Philadelphia hospital, he had access to everything that medicine could offer. As a last resort, he went on a macrobiotic program and totally cleared his cancer and his metastasis. (His before and after x-rays were published in LIFE magazine to prove his cure. Then he stopped the diet, his cancer recurred and he died.)

Elaine Nussbaum, (author of **RECOVERY,** Japan Publications, Kodansha International, Ltd. through Harper and Row Publishers, 10 East 53rd Street, New York, NY 10022, 1986), is a young mother in her thirties who developed cancer of the ovaries. This was, needless to say, the biggest shock of her life. But she geared up for it and ate as healthfully as possible, did everything she could with positive imagery and had a wonderful family support system behind her. In spite of all this, she continued to decline, as she had radiation treatments and chemotherapy. She was weakened, nauseated and bald.

Eventually her ovarian cancer spread to her lungs and liver and even the vertebral bodies of her back bone. The metastatic cancer caused her spine to collapse and left her in a wheelchair, hairless, withered, ridden with pain and incapacitated. She, likewise, wrote about her victory over cancer with the macrobiotic approach and has dissolved all of her cancer, and its metastases; her bones are healed and she is a practicing counselor this day (I lecture with her at the summer Kushi Institute conferences, and she is usually just coming in from jogging when I see her. She is exuberantly healthy and it is over 10 years).

When I read about these two cases, I figured, "Heck, if they can cure cancer, then E.I. ought to be a piece of cake". But I couldn't understand why it should be so beneficial, until I started researching the macrobiotic approach. Still there appeared to be so many drawbacks to macrobiotics that I put this information on the back shelf and pursued detoxification as the route to wellness. But further remarkable successes brought me back. The result has been this book, **YOU ARE WHAT YOU ATE** to get you started, then **THE CURE IS IN THE KITCHEN** to give you the intimate details of the strict healing phase that people used to heal the impossible. **TIRED OR TOXIC?** has over 33 explanations of why and how the macrobiotic diet has been able to heal the impossible. **WELLNESS AGAINST ALL ODDS** gives even more pearls for healing the impossible as well as for solutions for those who hate or cannot tolerate macro. **DEPRESSION CURED AT LAST!** takes you even further. There is continual growth and the more you want to be well, the more you will need to read.

CHAPTER III

NUTRITION:

DO YOU HAVE
THE VULNERABILITY FACTOR?

DON'T TOUCH THOSE VITAMINS

It's no secret that many myopic members of the medical profession are on a warpath against vitamins and recommend that lay people do not take them. In fact, they go so far as to state that the American diet provides all the nutrition that the average person needs. I made a search of the literature myself, to find that there are scores of papers proving marked mineral and vitamin deficiencies in many countries, including our own, and extending to all ages of our population. Here is just a minute sample regarding one of scores of nutrients, zinc:

Elsborg, in a study of 403 elderly Danes residing in their own homes, showed that zinc intake was low in 87% of the people. Holden showed that 68% of 22 American men and women eating self-selected diets were found to consume less than two-thirds of the RDA of zinc, while Cambridge showed that pregnant women ingested only about two-thirds of the recommended daily dietary allowance. The studies go on and on.

Most likely the same physicians and dietitians who recommend no vitamins are also the ones who make biochemical blunders daily by recommending hydrogenated grocery store corn oils and margarines for those with elevated cholesterols, thereby increasing their intakes of trans fatty acids, which actually stress the body chemistry and accelerate degenerative diseases (see the **E.I. SYNDROME, REVISED**). This same mind set supports the ingestion of processed foods which contain inferior levels of vitamins E, B6, and minerals like zinc and magnesium. These deficiencies coupled with the trans fatty acids push degeneration or deterioration (aging) even faster.

We did a study of over 400 people who consecutively reported to our office for diagnosis and management of allergic and environmentally induced illnesses (E.I.), and over 50 percent of these people had a zinc deficiency. Over a third of the others who were not deficient were marginally just above the lowest level of normal.

Upon studying the comments made by doctors opposed to nutritional supplementation, I finally figured out how physicians can confidently assert that vitamins are not needed.

1. They do not study the biochemistry literature to learn of the astounding flood of evidence for supplementation for a variety of conditions, and they do not seek out the literature to learn that their claims of nutritional adequacy are not substantiated; nor do they initiate their own studies. In other words, ignorance is bliss.

2. They don't realize that symptoms of nutritional deficiencies are subtle. Medicine is excellent at diagnosing end stage disease such as diabetes or hepatitis where grossly abnormal functions of blood tests occur. However, long before blood test abnormalities present themselves, people have symptoms. It's the early warning symptoms like chronic tiredness that alert one to find a

cause before end-stage organ failure occurs.

Unfortunately tests like the chemical profile that is drawn as part of an annual physical examination, are not sensitive enough to show abnormalities at the early stage of disease. Therefore, absence of blood test abnormality is assumed to mean absence of disease, an absolutely erroneous assumption. Medicine goes one step further labeling people who complain of these early symptoms as hypochondriacs, whereas in reality there is no such thing as a hypochondriac. If a person complains of something, even it is all in his head, it's the job of a physician to find out why he is complaining and try to help him. Therefore, no complaint is without merit, nor should it be ignored.

3. Oftentimes, physicians are put off by the claims of individuals recovering from vitamin deficiencies. In other words, they'll hear that vitamin B6 cleared one person's PMS, another person's depression, another person's fatigue, and another person's carpal tunnel syndrome. So they erroneously assume, having just graduated from the school of cookbook medicine, that B6 deficiency can't cause any of those symptoms. In essence, however, B6 is crucial in over 30 enzyme systems and not everyone, because of biochemical individuality, shorts the same enzymes. Therefore, different symptoms can occur. Zinc, for example, is crucial in over 90 enzymes. One person may short enzymes 1-5, another may short enzymes 50-55, and another may short another set of enzymes. Clearly, they will all have totally different symptoms.

And we can't blame the current state of the art entirely, for the patient shares some of the burden. Many people with nutritional deficiencies, because they have occurred so slowly, don't appreciate how bad they really feel. They have become used to feeling below par as a way of life. When an astute physician elicits minor symptoms, then hunts for, finds, and corrects the causative deficiencies, the patient experiences for the first time in years what feeling good is really all about. If you haven't felt good for many years, you tend to make many rationalizations and assume it's just part of stress or getting older. But as many people have told us, after their nutritional deficiencies were corrected, they hadn't felt so good in years. And in some cases, they had never felt so good, ever before.

Others have learned to ignore or tune-out early warning symptoms because they fear being labeled as hypochondriacs. Because we operate with a medical system that is not designed to diagnose and treat early body malfunction, we as physicians tend to label people as hypochondriacs and crocks when we can't find a cause for their complaints. This helps us save face.

4. Physicians fail to consider that just because the blood level for a nutrient falls within the "normal range", that this may not necessarily mean that this is the normal level for this particular person.

There is a vast difference between normal and optimal. Many of the values derived for nutritional supplements are drawn from a number of people who are not necessarily optimally healthy or feeling their best. For example, the normal level of B12 is 200-900. That's a tremendous range when you realize other levels, such as thyroid are much smaller. This suggests that many people at the lower end of the scale were not at optimal health. And it also suggests that if the range of normal is so huge, then how do we know that one particular individual's best level of function isn't 900 or even more, say 1200?

5. Opponents of vitamins argue that many of the vitamins are toxic and dangerous. This is true, but everything in the world is toxic or dangerous at some particular dose, including air and water. Everything has a bell-shaped curve of maximum desired effect.

But with a knowledge of human biochemistry and periodic monitoring of levels, how dangerous can a program be? Proclaiming danger is merely a way of covering up for lack of knowledge. Wouldn't it be more honest to simply refer to a specialist who does have special knowledge in nutritional biochemistry instead of denying the existence of untested deficiencies? That would be like me saying that no one needs a brain surgeon, since I don't know anything about doing brain surgery.

And once a nutrient deficiency is identified, it must be corrected. Understandably, there is a tremendous difference between corrective levels and maintenance levels of nutrients. Corrective levels are necessarily unbalanced to balance or correct an imbalance (the deficiency) in a person's chemistry that was identified through blood or urine tests. Then, after a few months, when the corrections have been made and monitored, a maintenance dosage can be employed, which is much lower and is, of necessity, a much more balanced scheme of nutrients.

For example, in correcting over 500 patients with abnormally low levels of RBC (red blood cell) zinc, I was amazed to find that 2 and 3 times the RDA (Recommended Daily Allowance) of 15 mg/day of zinc did not correct many people over a

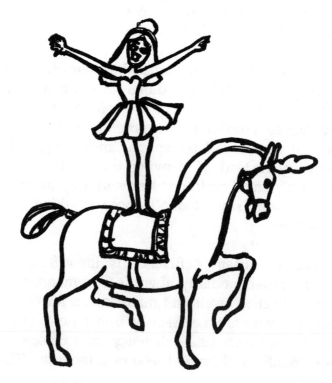

Correcting a nutritional deficiency requires quite a balancing act. Some physicians do not have the biochemical knowledge to do it. For example, they would not know that incorrectly correcting your zinc can cause deficiencies in copper, magnesium, manganese, molybdenum, and more.

period of two months. Many required levels of 90 mg or over. This is potentially dangerous because such extremely high levels can lower copper, molybdenum and manganese.

I, for one, was a conventionally trained physician who, for years, suffered exhaustion for no reason and kept looking through all of my medical textbooks to try to find a reason. One of the final answers was that I had multiple nutritional deficiencies, many of which could not be corrected until I had identified further hidden nutritional deficiencies.

For example, my vitamin A level was extremely low; I had eczema, so I had probably used it up prematurely with faster than normal skin repair. The result of a vitamin A deficiency is poor mucosal barrier integrity, which in turn made me more vulnerable to Candida. Anyway, after large doses of vitamin A, my level was not corrected. It wasn't until I found that I was zinc deficient that I could correct my vitamin A level. For you see, zinc is crucial in the enzyme alcohol dehydrogenase, which converts the primary form of vitamin A as retinol, into the first metabolic breakdown step of retinaldehyde. Without sufficient levels of the zinc dependent enzyme, alcohol hydrogenase, I could take vitamin A until I grew gills and it would not raise my level. And if I had measured the wrong test, a serum zinc instead of an RBC or erythrocyte zinc, I would not have found the zinc deficiency at all. Likewise even intravenous magnesium administration wouldn't correct my erythrocyte magnesium deficiency which manifested itself as months of intolerable back spasm in an area of old injury, until I had discovered and corrected my manganese deficiency. And on and on it went. Each nutrient is dependent upon other nutrients as well as a healthy gut if correction of nutrient deficiencies is going to occur.

So you see, not only is the field of nutrition complex, but one undetected deficiency can lead to another, which in turn leads to increased vulnerability for various disease states. In other words, it snowballs or spreads.

This domino effect of one deficiency leading to another, most likely contributes to the spreading phenomenon of E.I. The spreading phenomenon occurs when the victim starts reacting to more and more things that never bothered him before. The mechanism is partly due to an accumulation or backlog of chemicals being presented to a nutritionally incomplete detoxification system.

This completely baffles the physician untrained in nutritional biochemistry and environmental medicine because what he sees is a person with over a dozen vague complaints of exhaustion, feeling "unreal" or spacey and depressed for no reason. These patients also have a half dozen recognizable complaints like migraines, chronic sinusitis, spastic colon, arthralgia, or asthma.

On top of this, all the exams, x-rays, and blood tests are normal. And to make matters worse, as the patient snowballs further, he starts reacting to things that never before bothered him—various foods, stores, cigarette smoke, cleansers, constructions glues, new carpets and more.

Then the last straw comes when the spreading phenomenon has reached its peak and he reacts faster and more vigorously to these triggers. By this time, everyone, including the patient is left doubting the sanity of the patient; and only because modern medicine is not well-versed in the molecular biology and biochemistry of **the spreading phenomenon**.

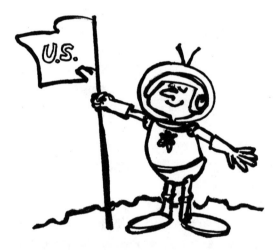

If we can put a man on the moon, it seems that we should routinely look at his vitamin and mineral levels.

A typical scenario is a young woman who gets hooked on sweets, colas and processed foods. She gets married, starts taking the birth control pill and smoking. As she gets more depleted of nutrients, she gets colds more easily and is put on antibiotics. As she feels more drained, she has more coffee and sweets in an attempt to increase her energy. Then she gets recurrent vaginal infections and starts with intestinal symptoms of gas, bloating, and indigestion. Her childhood hay-fever symptoms of chronic headaches, and postnasal drip re-surface and she slowly descends to constant tiredness and unwarranted depression. She may have a pregnancy, root canal, auto accident, severe psychological stress such as a divorce, or move into a new house or renovated office. Soon she starts reacting with symptoms to various foods, chemicals, molds, but all medical exams are fruitless and life seems to be coming to a halt. At this stage she has full-blown environmental illness or E.I., that believe it or not, can get much worse than this.

The treatment? Simple. We just reverse the unhealthy processes of the 21st century.

We look for hidden vitamin and mineral deficiencies. We put her on a diet of no sweets, no processed foods, heavy in greens, whole grains, seeds, beans, root vegetables and sometimes mineral-rich seaweeds. We treat the Candida problem. We test her for hidden mold sensitivities and treat them. It's a rare victim who isn't loaded with them. We have her adopt a chemically less-contaminated lifestyle by getting rid of smelly cleansers, fragrant cosmetics and toiletries, old carpets, use air purification devices and more. Later we can test for hidden food and chemical sensitivities if needed.

In essence, we whittle away at her total 21st century body

burden or load (as we described in **THE E.I. SYNDROME, REVISED**), until she is unloaded enough to heal and feel better than she has ever remembered.

Most likely, in years to come, medicine will no longer rely on such gross tests of end organ failure as the chemical profile, such as it exists today. Most likely, we will draw a few tubes of blood and be able to assay within minutes your every vitamin, mineral, essential fatty acid, and amino acid. Until that time, we have to continue doing blood assays as money (insurance companies seem to harbor a particular disdain for nutrient levels) and availability of specific tests permit. A few pieces of the puzzle are far better than no pieces at all.

ARE YOU A NUTRITIONAL TIME BOMB WAITING TO GO OFF?

When every doctor has been stumped, after all the blood tests and x-rays come back negative and yet still you are caught in a maze of seemingly unrelated symptoms, even you will begin to doubt your own sanity. Most likely you have the vulnerability factor: an unrecognized nutritional deficiency.

Everyone was excited about the face-lift that the office was getting. New pastel paints were chosen, a lovely beige carpet was glued down, new draperies and chairs and artificial potted plants were added. It was about time that the old office had some renovations. As the work continued, however, one person became progressively sicker.

Gina at first started having headaches, then she found she couldn't concentrate. She was depressed for no reason. When she got home in the evening she was so exhausted she could

35

think of nothing except going straight to bed. Slowly other symptoms started. Every time she ate chocolate she would have a severe headache. This had never happened before.

Every time she went back into the building she could smell the glues and the paints and the new carpet. She asked her coworkers if it bothered them, but everybody just looked at her as through she were a little strange. She went to her doctor finally to have a good physical and he gave her a clean bill of health.

After a while she started getting extremely nauseated; she just could no longer concentrate. She went to several other doctors and again was told that everything was fine. With time she began to doubt her own sanity. For after all, everyone else was happy in the new office and she was the only one reacting. If there was something in there, surely other people would be involved. And if there was something wrong with her, surely one of the six physicians that she eventually saw would have found it. The reason they didn't however, is that Gina is one of the myriads of people who have E.I. or Environmental Illness. And out of over half a million physicians in the United States there are less than 400 physicians who have passed the oral and written board examinations of the American Academy of Environmental Medicine, and who are trained in diagnosing and treating environmental illness.

One of the first things we found in Gina's blood work-up was that her red blood cell (RBC) zinc was abnormally low. This is most likely one of the factors that made her so vulnerable. For when the zinc becomes low, the body is not able to detoxify chemicals as quickly. Zinc is crucial in over a dozen pathways in the detoxification mechanism of the liver.

Normally the liver is constantly at work detoxifying the chemicals that are in food, air and water. But when a zinc deficiency is present, one major detoxification enzyme, alcohol dehydrogenase, can suffer. This is the primary enzyme for the breakdown (or detoxication or biotransformation) of many chemicals.

When this enzyme is no longer functional, the chemicals must find a different pathway to follow. Take trichloroethylene. It is found in many people's blood streams from the dry cleaning fluid in their clothes and carpets, glues and construction adhesives at home and at work, as well as in the drinking water in most municipalities as an industrial contaminant. It is also used to decaffeinate coffee. As a prevalent solvent, it is widespread in its use in the United States.

Chemicals can enter the blood through the lungs. All things that you breathe or smell can get into the blood and brain. Once in the blood, they take a pass through the liver, since this is one of nature's check points to help keep us clear of poisons and toxins. Once they enter the liver to be detoxified, there isn't just one pathway, but sometimes as many as a dozen different routes a chemical can take. The route that is taken depends on which route is available and which ones are already taken and busy detoxifying other chemicals that got there first.

When the alcohol dehydrogenase pathway is blocked, as in a zinc deficiency, one of the breakdown or detox pathways a chemical can take leads to the formation of chloral hydrate. You may remember this name as the old "Mickey Finn" or knock-out drops, which cause exactly the same symptoms that people with environmental illness experience:

37

tremendous exhaustion, dizziness, nausea, inability to concentrate, spaciness, numbness and tingling in the extremities, mood swings and much more.

Detoxification pathways can be weakened in two ways: they can be overloaded by too many other chemicals or they can be improperly functioning due to nutrient deficiencies. When this happens, chemicals that before never bothered a person, now start giving him symptoms. He can no longer tolerate cigarette smoke, or perfumes or certain stores, or the smell of certain cleansers and he can have headaches or dizziness or nausea or cough triggered by each exposure.

When the detoxification system is ailing (from chemical exposure overload and/or nutrient deficiencies), subsequent chemicals from daily exposures get backed up in the blood. Without enough minerals in the detoxification enzymes, chemical exposures that never before bothered someone will now cause alarming reactions that seem out of proportion or distorted. To compound the problem, the responses are not consistent from one exposure time to the next due to many factors: (1) shifting of pathway availability as the body attempts to cope with the overload, and (2) the total body burden which is never the same at any two moments in time. In other words, if minerals are missing in one path, the body may shift detox responsibility to another path. But if this one is busy detoxifying something else, then it shifts to another. But each path may give different symptoms. So you may not have the same symptom from the same exposure or trigger. To the observer, it really looks like the person reacting is a hypochondriac. And the bewildered reactor is left not even able to think rationally, much less figure out what is happening.

For example the morning you have coffee and a donut for breakfast and get caught in heavy traffic, may be the day that you get a headache and mood swings from the newly glued baseboard molding in the office. Whereas on a day when you have spent the weekend in fresh air and had a healthful breakfast, the glue doesn't bother you.

With a build up of chemicals in the blood, cell membranes are attacked and become weak. Chemicals enter the cell easily and damage further regulatory chemistry. The brain membranes and cells are particularly vulnerable. Also, the intracellular mitochondrial membranes which are responsible for energy synthesis are easily damaged. So inability to concentrate and exhaustion mysteriously emerge.

SO LET'S SEE WHAT DAMAGE A DEFICIENCY IN JUST ONE NUTRIENT CAN DO

An undiscovered zinc deficiency can lead to poor absorption and metabolism of other nutrients. For example, zinc is of primary importance in an enzyme called carbonic anhydrase, which is responsible for making the gastric (stomach) hydrochloric acid or HCL which is crucial for absorption of minerals. Alcohol dehydrogenase is a zinc dependent enzyme necessary for the absorption of vitamin A. You can take vitamin A in extremely high doses and never correct a deficiency of it, if you do not have sufficient alcohol dehydrogenase enzyme to convert vitamin A from retinol to retinaldehyde, its first breakdown step.

Pyridoxine kinase is an important zinc enzyme, which facilitates the breakdown of vitamin B6 to its first usable step, pyridoxal-5-phosphate. This goes on to be necessary in the synthesis of all brain neurotransmitters or chemicals that are responsible for our moods. You can begin to see how a deficiency of one single mineral can spread into a maze of symptoms which confuse the physician untrained in environmental and nutritional medicine.

Zinc enzymes are necessary for proper insulin storage. Does this relate to the high incidence of hypoglycemia symptoms seen in E.I.? Zinc is crucial in DNA polymerase, an enzyme that keeps our genetics stable. Does this explain why after a particular chemical exposure we were suddenly different, never to return to totally normal non-sensitive beings again? Dr. Barbara McClintock received the Nobel Prize (1983) thirty years after she discovered that genes can change in response to an organism's attempt to adapt to a foreign environment. Without proper enzymes to control the "jumping genes" as they are called, they are more prone to distortion or re-arrangement. The result can be a new program: that of the monster called E.I.

Zinc and taurine form a conjugate that protects cell membranes. Is this why people with E.I. are prone to fluid retention, crazy mood swings (brain swelling), exhaustion, cardiac arrhythmia (when it feels like your heart is doing cartwheels), and chemical sensitivity? It's highly likely since these are all phenomena of sick or defective membranes. With deficient zinc, the cell membranes are left naked or vulnerable to attack by chemicals. (And more chemicals are spilling over into the blood because the liver is less able to handle them when it's zinc-dependent detoxification enzymes are suffering). When chemicals attack membranes, they develop holes and leaks. The leaky cell behaves abnormally and the symptoms are determined by which organs' cells suffer the most.

40

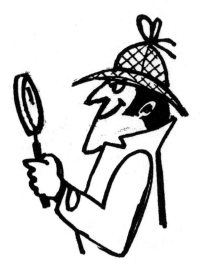

Finding one nutritional deficiency is a clue that there are others. It's very unlikely that a person can develop a singular biochemical deficiency.

If brain cells are leaky, you get all the crazy mental symptoms, spacey, etc. If it's heart cells, you get palpitations, if it's blood vessel cells, you get swelling, hypertension, lupus, or vasculitis. If it's liver mitochondrial walls, you have poor energy, or chronic fatigue.

Many types of saran type plastics (vinylidene chlorides) are metabolized into aldehydes, as are many rubber products. Candida toxicity can also produce aldehydes, as do many environmental pollutants, such as exhaust fumes and formaldehyde from myriads of home and office furnishings. These aldehydes can mimic some of the tremendous brain fog, or inability to concentrate, exhaustion, poor memory and dizziness so classic in chemically intolerant people. They can also proceed to contribute to the chemistry that produces cancer years later. Carbonic anhydrase is a zinc dependent enzyme which has to do with buffering of this acetaldehyde and the metabolism of it. Obviously if zinc is deficient in this enzyme, there is reason for further accentuation of the severe depression and brain fog, which is so commonly seen in victims of E.I.

So what am I saying? If zinc is deficient in just **one** enzyme, for example carbonic anhydrase, the body can start reacting to Candida, exhaust fumes and buildings. The chief target organ is usually the brain, and the most common symptoms are spaciness and difficulty concentrating. If zinc is deficient in another enzyme (alcohol dehydrogenase), the spreading phenomenon can occur. If it's deficient in other enzymes, there is abnormal gene repair, vitamin metabolism, enzyme synthesis, membrane integrity, etc.

Now, recall zinc is only one mineral and is in over 90 enzymes. I've only given you a brief sketch of the symptoms

42

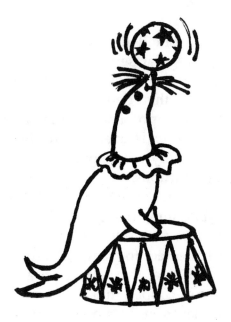

To balance one's nutrients requires:

1. Excellent biochemical guidance.
2. Reduction in chemical load and improvement in diet (the two things that probably caused it in the first place).
3. Periodic assessment, since nothing that is alive is a static phenomenon.

that 5 of those enzymes could produce if someone were zinc deficient. You can clearly see that a hidden zinc deficiency can be the perfect set-up for developing chemical sensitivities, as well as the emergence of other sensitivities to pollens, dusts, molds, foods, Candida, and additional chemicals. This spreading phenomenon creates the **universal reactor**, sensitive to everything.

In order to check for a zinc deficiency, however, a physician must be aware that a regular serum zinc will not suffice. A special test of red blood cell or erythrocyte zinc is the test of choice that will show this deficiency. Correction of the deficiency is not without problems either. In treating well over 500 patients with zinc deficiencies, we have seen that it must be done very carefully with a great deal of appreciation for its biochemical interactions.

For example, molybdenum, manganese, copper and other minerals can all displace each other from crucial enzymes. If a zinc deficiency is treated too aggressively or incorrectly without the proper balance, the patient, in a month or two, will have deficiencies of copper, molybdenum, or manganese. These in turn have their own lists of voluminous symptoms. For example, copper is in over a dozen enzymes. A copper deficiency might affect the enzyme ascorbic acid dehydrogenase, so that one cannot break down vitamin C or ascorbic acid into its first usable metabolite.

Another facet that came from this research was that in most people, very high levels of zinc were required to correct deficiencies slowly over several months. No one would dream of using, for example, levels of zinc ten times the normal RDA without having blood tests available to monitor not only the progress of the zinc, but that of the copper, manganese and other minerals that can be involved in this delicate balance.

In the beginning when a correction is begun, levels are necessarily unbalanced, since the individual is already unbalanced with his deficiency. Later on when the correction has been made, and the balance can be checked in the blood, then maintenance levels of nutrients can be prescribed, which have a far different balance than a corrective prescription. If the corrective prescription is taken beyond the prescribed time, the pendulum swings to the opposite side and imbalance results in other nutrients.

We are entering an era where doctors will need to start learning molecular biochemistry and the science of nutrition. For due to the over-work of the body's chemical detoxification system from our 21st century diets and lifestyles, many people are nutritional time bombs just waiting to go off. They're missing many nutrients and are in a poor state of balance and no one knows it. They themselves know that something is wrong, though, and that they are not playing with a full deck (of nutrients). But they don't know how to go about finding the solution. E.I. is a product of the 21st century and it shows us that many rules of medicine are inadequately archaic. When one is already chemically overloaded, you can't treat him by giving another chemical or drug.

Many of them (like myself) will, or have, gone on to become victims of environmental illness, with reactivity to dusts, molds, pollens, Candida, foods, and many chemicals. But by correcting their nutritional deficiencies they can strengthen their detoxification enzymes once again, and come out even healthier than they have ever been.

How does one know if he might be a nutritional time bomb waiting to go off? Very easily. Many already sense that they do not feel vivacious, happy and enthusiastic the majority of the time. They know that there is something wrong. That is the time to find themselves an environmentally and nutritionally oriented physician, before their time bomb goes off.

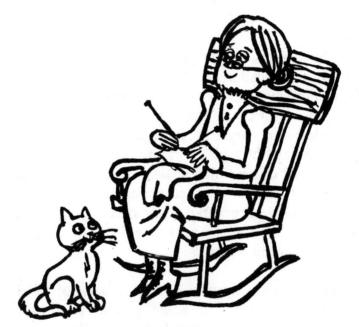

Even Granny knew a stitch in time saves nine. It makes sense to identify nutritional deficiencies when symptoms are nebulous and minor.

CHAPTER IV

DETOXICATION:

THE PATH TO REJUVENATION

FOR DOCTORS ONLY. This chapter is too technical for the average reader. Most may want to skim through the technical parts and get on with their program. Later on, curiosity may spur you to return to it in more depth.

As you have seen, the body has a vast xenobiotic (foreign chemical) detoxication (also called biotransformation or detoxification) system. Major in the liver, it extends through the lungs, gastrointestinal tract, skin, and kidneys, metabolizing and excreting foreign chemicals that enter the body every day through contaminated air, food and water. This xenobiotic detoxication system requires a vast amount of energy and nutrients to function maximally. Although the body can heal a surprising array of wounds, diseases and broken bones, as well as broken spirits, it needs optimum health for optimum wellness.

Rejuvenation, or an apparent turning back of the hands of time, definitely occurs in some people as they begin to depurate, or unload accumulated toxins that accelerate the chemistry of aging. Everyone has a particular load of toxins that is so individual that it's like a biochemical fingerprint. These toxins can be reduced, thereby reducing the stress to the body. Likewise in order to heal many conditions, an unloading is necessary.

For example, in some cases, people with E.I. cannot improve past a certain point using a good ecologic program because their cellular biochemistry or machinery has been poisoned. These poisons simply must be removed before healing can progress.   These poisons can be old drugs, pesticides, medicines, or many of the thousands of chemicals we are exposed to daily in our food, air, and water. Whatever their sources, whatever their routes of contamination (absorbed through skin, lungs, or gut), once they are in the body, chemicals can act like a monkey wrench in a cogwheel, impeding normal function until they are removed. And a poorly functioning chemistry makes one a more easy prey to disease and speeds up deterioration or aging.

The body has many ways of getting rid of these chemicals or detoxifying the body. (Incidentally, in science, this is more properly called detoxication or biotransformation, and foreign chemicals in the body are termed xenobiotics. At first I hesitated using such big words, but they are words you will hear in the future anyway. PCB's, dioxin and radon were unfamiliar ten years ago, but everyone has some glimmer of what they connote today. Likewise, xenobiotic detoxication will roll off your lips in the future, so you might as well begin to practice.) Anyway, once a chemical has gained entry to the body, it can undergo a variety of chemical reactions in the body's attempt to get rid of it. There are many possible pathways, some good and some harmful.

Sometimes the body goofs and turns the chemical into a more dangerous or even more carcinogenic (cancer-causing) chemical.   Sometimes the body has a dozen possible pathways that can be used, but chooses a particular one because the other paths are already overloaded detoxifying other chemicals that got there first. Later on it may use some of these alternate pathways and produce totally different metabolites than it did initially, and some of them are more

49

dangerous than the initial, or parent, compound.

Obviously, if on one occasion you're exposed to form-aldehyde, for example, and it is metabolized quickly into a harmless chemical, you'll not react. But say on another day you had had some other exposures as well as your formaldehyde. The regular pathway might be overloaded, so the formaldehyde is shunted to a different route which produces metabolites that cross into the brain and produce depression. And this is a very simplified example of the total load. Imagine what happens as you inhale and ingest scores of toxic chemicals all day and night? Sometimes a chemical is so abnormal, the body doesn't have a good chemical setup to detoxify and it stays in the body, usually as a transformed metabolite.

The organs the body uses to expel chemicals are the lungs, skin, bowel, bladder, and reproductive organs. That's it. There are no other ways to get rid of chemicals. They have to exit from one of those places.

The liver is the most active organ in transforming these chemicals so that they can be expelled. In the cells of the liver are a series of membranes called the endoplasmic reticulum (ER) where a vast amount of this chemistry goes on. This chemistry is dependent on many nutrients in order to proceed. So it seemed logical to us to look at making a nutritional detoxication program. In other words, if the nutrients which the detox pathways depend upon are beefed up enough, this should facilitate the body in detoxifying itself even against greater 21st century environmental stresses. Such a program must be individualized to the person, however. There is no canned approach as we have available in much of medicine, because everyone is so unique.

To further complicate matters, nearly every nutrient plays a role in the detoxication process of xenobiotics. You've already seen how just one deficiency like zinc can affect every major biochemical pathway in the body, and that a deficiency of this one nutrient has far-reaching effects in terms of the body's ability or disability to detoxify. There is also a domino effect whereby its persistent lack is felt in many enzyme systems that themselves go on to further disturb other enzymes, causing many other deficiencies.

Likewise, a deficiency of zinc in the xenobiotic detoxication system causes a buildup of chemicals in the liver which can further damage and stress the already ailing detoxification system. It's sort of like the branching of a tree. If one element is missing, then several other pathways are secondarily adversely effected, and then these pathways furthermore effect changes in numerous other pathways. And what is the result? The snowballing or spreading phenomenon we have so frequently seen that results in the universal reactor, or those who react to everything: molds (which includes Candida), foods and chemicals.

One of the worse symptoms the universal reactor endures is the **toxic brain syndrome**. He feels exhausted, can't concentrate, spacey, dizzy, nauseated, and headachy. He feels like he has been drugged; and to complicate this nightmare, there are few blood tests or x-rays to diagnose it.

To further complicate matters, the toxic brain syndrome is not caused by just one or two things. The cumulative triggers can include such things as an unsuspected nutritional deficiency, an emotional strain, or a heightened sensitivity to molds, food, Candida, and chemicals as well as by many other things.

We are now beginning to understand some of the biochemical mechanisms of it. Some of the most common problems are indoor and outdoor chemicals, such as the hydrocarbons. Not a day goes by where you are not exposed to these at home, at work, or in your food or water. We are beginning to learn how these 21st century foreign chemicals broadly known in the biological world as xenobiotics, can cause **brain fog** or toxic brain syndrome.

Common xenobiotics, or foreign chemicals, include such hydrocarbons as xylene, benzene, toluene, vinyl chloride, and trichloroethylene (TCE). These are the chemicals found in plastics, glues, paints, clothing, furnishings, food and water.

Because these hydrocarbons are lipid soluble, and the brain has a greater affinity for absorbing fat-soluble (lipid) materials than do other tissues, the brain gets higher levels of these toxins. This explains why the brain is one of the primary target organs and why baffling brain symptoms predominate. We call these cerebral symptoms, **brain fog** or toxic brain syndrome.

The liver, the main detoxifying organ in the body, contains certain specialized cellular components (microsomes), which participate in metabolizing foreign chemicals (xenobiotics). These cellular components process the foreign chemicals so that they can eventually be eliminated from the body. Of course these microsomes are made of membranes, so as chemicals accumulate, also in these lipid membranes, the very membranes that are responsible for detox get damaged. You can now appreciate the complexity of the spreading phenomenon and how difficult it is to arrest.

Xenobiotics, in the course of being metabolized, undergo

several chemical changes (oxidations, reductions, degradations, and conjugations). Most of the time they are made less toxic, but occasionally they are made more toxic. Oftentimes a single chemical will have many metabolites. In other words, the xenobiotic can be broken down into a dozen different chemical compounds each with its own selective actions and side effects. (I hesitated to make some of these repetitions, but then I reminded myself that you're learning molecular biochemistry and toxicology concepts that many physicians do not know. Hence, some repetition of sophisticated concepts should reinforce the learning process painlessly.)

The ability of the body to degrade (change or reduce) these chemicals depends on how many other chemicals the body is exposed to at the same time from contaminated air, food, and water. Prescription drugs and radiation also add to the burden by creating free radicals that damage membranes. It is the combination or total load and genetic factors that determine how well the body handles the additional chemicals.

The nutritional state of the individual's detoxification enzyme system and the availability of certain selected nutrients, including essential lipids, and amino acids, also affect the ability of the body to break down these foreign chemicals.

TRICHLOROETHYLENE AS AN EXAMPLE

Take trichloroethylene for example. It is an all-purpose xenobiotic and, like formaldehyde, is difficult to avoid in everyday living. It is widely used in industry and is an intermediary of many chemical reactions.

It is an anesthetic, a degreaser, a dry cleaning fluid, an intermediary of plastics, oils, glues, and a common drinking water contaminant. It is one of the "inert ingredients" of pesticides, and is even used in the food industry to decaffeinate coffee and tea.

TCE, like many other xenobiotics, is broken down with the first pass through the liver into several by-products. One of these by-products is a chemical family called epoxides. Another metabolite is formic acid (formaldehyde), a potent toxin for most chemically sensitive individuals.

Then there are further pathways that epoxides can take. They can attach to DNA. When this happens, drastic changes may occur in our genetics which can result in mutation. It could also potentially cause the following: liver toxicity, kidney toxicity, brain toxicity, suppression of the immune system, teratogenesis (birth defects), environmental illness, accelerated aging, or even cancer.

Or other trichloroethylene by-products can attach to glutathione and eventually be excreted in the bile. Then again, other trichloroethylene by-products can be converted to aldehydes. Aldehydes are cell toxins which start the formation of free radicals, cross-linking, and membrane destruction. These three processes have to do with the chemistry of aging, chronic degenerative diseases and cancer.

Last, but not least, trichloroethylene can be converted into chloral hydrate, a hypnotic or sedative better known as "Mickey Finn" or "knock-out drops". In the **Physician's Desk Reference** (PDR, a book describing dosages and side effects of all prescription drugs), the list of side effects reads like any typical patient with environmental illness (E.I.). All

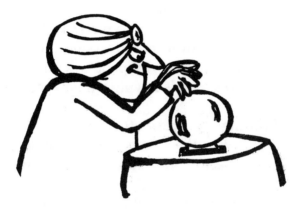

No one knows which biochemical pathway a particular chemical will take in your body on a specific day. In people whose detox systems are overloaded, common everyday chemicals often breakdown into substances toxic to the brain like chloral hydrate (the old "Mickey Finn").

the symptoms of brain fog are present plus peripheral neuropathy (numbness and tingling) and almost any other symptom you can think of.

CANDIDA AND DETOX

Remember, alcohol, inhaled chemicals and Candida add increased aldehyde. And in the brain, it can cause the toxic brain symptoms of E.I. (spaciness, dopiness, exhaustion, numbness and tingling, depression for no reason and more). So a drink of alcohol, for example, can put further stress on the detoxification mechanisms, and increase the acetaldehyde levels of an already compromised system and increase the Candida symptoms. That's why people with E.I. can't drink much, while everyone else is having a merry old time.

Candida, according to Truss' theory, raises acetaldehyde levels; Candida in the bowel can contribute to a malabsorption of specific nutrients, especially vitamin A, and increase levels of alanine which inhibit intracellular levels of cysteine (needed for further glutathione production which is necessary for detoxification). And so you begin to appreciate the tremendous chemical effect and why people with no training in the biochemistry of E.I. are baffled by our symptoms. But it all fits so beautifully. Look at the hundreds of people who became less chemically sensitive as soon as they treated their Candida. They merely began to reduce their total load or total body burden. And thereby stop the snow balling or exponential worsening.

To reiterate, aldehyde production can come from many sources: trichloroethylene, alcohol, and Candida, as well as many other aldehyde precursors such as auto exhaust,

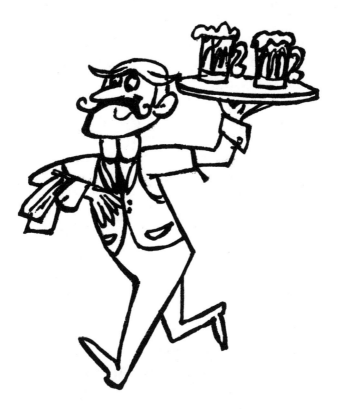

Alcohol is just another chemical that stresses the detox pathways. It breaks down to form aldehydes which are also formed from formaldehyde, auto exhaust, and vinylidene chloride (saran wrap, plastics). So no wonder people with E.I. can get blitzed so easily!

formaldehyde, etc.

Therefore, as you can see, understanding the biochemistry of detoxification helps one to understand the symptoms of E.I., for they are one.

IMPORTANT NUTRIENTS OF DETOX PATHWAYS

With all this happening, it's not surprising that people with E.I. feel like they are drugged; a wise person will begin to ask himself, is he tired or toxic? Many are really toxic; poisoned by 21st century xenobiotics. But why does E.I. effect some and not others? How can susceptible people improve their detoxification systems to allow them to tolerate levels of xenobiotics? What are the crucial elements that make a difference?

The level of cell nutrition is an important factor. Detoxification systems in the body are extremely dependent upon optimal nutritional supplementation of vitamins, minerals, essential fatty acids, and amino acids in order to ensure efficient detoxification and at the same time ensure efficient energy production and cellular stability.

Particularly important nutritional compounds in this regard include the B vitamins, especially B3 and B5, taurine (an amino acid) and the anti-oxidants, vitamins A, C, E and selenium and the minerals, zinc, copper and magnesium. Dimethylglycine (DMG), phosphatidyl choline, and countless other nutrients are also important.

For some of the many nutritional supplements required for detoxification, their specific uses for particular detoxification functions follows. In places, it does become technical, and I apologize as we struggle to make complicated biochemistry understandable for everyone. Your health depends on it.

The enzyme system NADPH is very active in changing chemicals to less dangerous forms that can be excreted and is extremely dependent upon high levels of vitamin B3 (niacin). However an alarming reaction can occur if one uses it without guidance (see **THE E.I. SYNDROME, REVISED**). Acetaldehyde toxicity can occur with Candida problems and chemical overload from plastics and formaldehyde, for example, requires good levels of taurine, zinc, and B5 (pantothenic acid) to stabilize cell membranes; and aldehyde oxidase which is necessary to further metabolize acetaldehyde (a major cause of brain fog) requires molybdenum.

Since glutathione carries chemicals out of the liver and into the bile, taurine, essential fatty acids, and B5 again are needed to improve bile flow.

Mitochondrial membranes (which are the source of energy in the cell and are involved in protein synthesis and lipid metabolism) and endoplasmic reticulum membranes (structures that house the xenobiotic detoxifying microsomes) require phosphatidyl choline and phosphatidyl ethanolamine for their fluidity and function; they also need magnesium, vitamin A, beta-carotene, vitamin E, eicosapentaenoic acid (EPA), choline, and carnitine.

Of the anti-oxidants, vitamin A stabilizes cell and organelle membranes, while vitamin E grabs passing chemicals that attempt to enter the cell. Vitamin C is the only free-floating, general purpose anti-oxidant vitamin that is extra cellular (that is, it is outside of the cell protecting against xenobiotics). The rest are intracellular or inside enzymes.

Glutathione peroxidase, which helps to keep microsomal and other membrane lipids in a less toxic state, requires selenium, vitamin E, and cysteine. Glutathione reductase must have healthy levels of B2 in order to function; and liver regeneration and generation metabolism are dependent upon thiamine or vitamin B1 (as acetaldehyde and free radicals attempt to weaken and damage the liver).

Formic acid metabolism (formaldehyde) relies heavily on folic acid (a B vitamin) and aldehyde dehydrogenase (an enzyme that may require molybdenum to function).

The superoxide dismutases are the body's "anti-arthritis" enzymes and protect against free radical attack that produces the aching of arthritis. They must have sufficient zinc and copper; while the mitochondrial superoxide dismutase contains manganese. And, of course, high levels of manganese must be present in order for magnesium to be absorbed, which itself is in over 300 enzymes and pathways in the body.

These are just a few of the nutritional supplements that are required for a healthy detoxification system.

It's also important to keep in mind that the detoxification system is not isolated. The way individuals see the world around them determines the way the body functions. **Attitude** affects the modulation of brain neuro-transmitters with in turn have an effect on the immune system, the acid/alkaline balance, the endocrine system, and the detoxication system. A healthy attitude is vital to a healthy body.

This is one reason why immunologists, internists, endocrinologists, and allergists are not able to identify and study the problems of E.I. They study isolated aspects of body physiology and rely on information that can be reproduced in test tubes. The problem is that there is no test tube that contains all the interrelated aspects of the body. The field of environmental medicine possesses **no artificial boundaries** and does not restrict itself to biochemistry or neurology, or immunology.

It's ironic that it's illegal to drive under the heavy influence of marijuana, alcohol, and drugs like chloral hydrate, but it's okay to drive in a new vinyl interior car behind a diesel truck. And it's OK to stop at the local dry cleaners and tank up directly on trichloroethylene. In the susceptible individual these all cause brain fog. The presence of trichloroethylene is measurable in the blood for several hours after a five minute visit to the dry cleaners. And, of course, wearing a newly dry cleaned suit keeps these levels going all day, as does working in an environment where this has been used to clean the carpets.

References in the biochemistry literature abound which support the above information, but because scientific disciplines are so fragmented, biochemists are rarely called upon to treat E.I. victims, and physicians rarely have enough time to read the journals in their own fields, much less those in nutrition, biochemistry, toxicology, and environmental medicine. But the mechanisms and scientific references for all of this are made clear in **TIRED OR TOXIC?**

Fortunately, it has been possible to detox people by

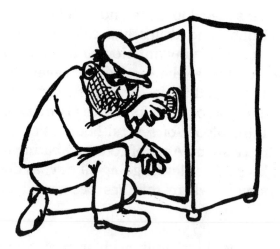

One of the secrets to getting well is to get rid of stored chemicals and detoxify. Macrobiotics appears to be one such method of accomplishing this.

improving their nutrition. Ailing chemistry can be corrected and even pushed to maximize the detox pathways.

After this, if xenobiotics persist, there are medically supervised sauna programs where chemicals can actually be sweated out. But often people returning from these programs had mineral and vitamin imbalances that had to be corrected, and they were not completely well.

But there are other methods through which the body can **discharge toxins.** Macrobiotics is one. Most of the persistent or stored chemicals are walled off in the fat. They must be mobilized (through exercise, sweating, weight loss, skin brushing): this turns them loose in the blood stream. Here they flow to all organs including the liver and the brain. The result is the person may feel very sick at this stage. It's here also that the liver must be in tip top shape to detoxify and excrete these chemicals to get rid of them quickly once and for all. It's best to enter into such a program knowing that the levels of crucial detoxication nutrients are in good balance. Get your vitamin and mineral levels assessed and corrected as soon as possible, as this will make the journey easier.

People going through macrobiotics will periodically experience a cleanse or discharge, where they will have a tender liver area, for example, and recurrence of some of their old symptoms. It's important at this point to try to avoid medication to suppress the symptoms (which adds to the chemical overload), but ride it out. Depending on the severity of symptoms however, close medical monitoring may be necessary. One may require blood tests at that time to be sure a discharge is being experienced, and not another sickness. We also can do extensive analyses of the vitamin, mineral, fatty acid, and amino acid levels to determine the state of biochemistry and correct it. Also, during the course of the program periodic checks should be made for biochemical balance to monitor and correct any serious deficiencies resulting from the stress on the detox system.

E.I. is a newcomer to the field of medicine and also to the discipline of macrobiotics. It breaks many rules. Ferments and grains are often not tolerated. Often detox is delayed because foreign chemicals, whether they be from mercury amalgams, pesticides, or inhaled chemicals, throw a monkey wrench in the mechanism. And thanks to the processed diet, many nutritional deficiencies further paralyze the detox process. But we are learning how to overcome much of this as we seek to eat and live closer to nature, instead of fighting her.

CURRENT MEDICAL THINKING IS OBSOLETE

Ecology and macrobiotics have much philosophy in common, leaving the viewpoint of "modern medicine" in the dark ages. Current disease concepts are definitely inadequate for wellness at many fundamental levels. They have served us well for years, but the time to march on has passed. The current thinking needs to adapt to the following concepts:

1. Failure is almost guaranteed with the **"victim" mentality**. The "Poor me, why did this have to happen to me?" leaves the person feeling powerless. Medicine further strengthens this concept of the powerless patient by having him visit a doctor-deity who has the power to prescribe chemicals with intimidating names to relieve symptoms.

In ecology and macrobiotics, YOU are responsible for your illness, as well as your wellness. YOU are the one who ate all the wrong foods and YOU are the only one who has the power to restore YOUR wellness and to help YOU reach new levels of wellness. YOU have all the power. How YOU use it is up to YOU.

2. Every symptom has a cause. In modern medicine, drugs are prescribed to cover up symptoms. In ecology and macrobiotics, the cause of symptoms is sought. The attention is directed at how the diet and lifestyle should be altered to allow nature's healing to take place. For example, millions of dollars worth of arthritis and colitis drugs are prescribed each year. But rare is the doctor who clears arthritis by identifying that beef, potato and natural gas are the triggers. Yet these are common causes.

3. **Biochemical individuality**. The modern doctor needs to abandon the cookbook formula: chief complaints, history, exam, blood test, x-ray, diagnosis, drug prescription or surgery. Medicine sees all diabetics as one person and all ulcers as one person. Hence, the cookbook approach.

When I was in medical school 30 years ago, when we would walk into a room for medical rounds, we wouldn't be walking in to see Mrs. Jones; we would be walking in to see the "gall bladder in #302". This results in a viewpoint that not only ignores biochemical individuality, but the individual himself! How can we even hope to successfully bring relief to a patient who possesses no individual identity?

Ecology recognizes that if you take 100 arthritics, every one of them is going to have a different cause. They will have

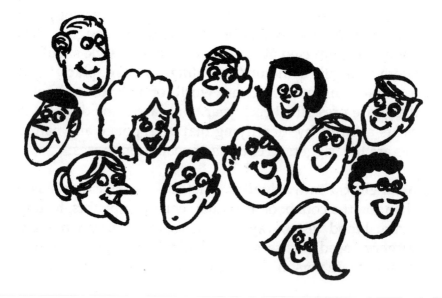

Cookbook medicine is very popular in the western world, where all people with arthritis, for example are presumed to have the same cause, since they all have the same disease. Hence, medicine is still searching for that elusive single cause.

Eastern medicine, however (for thousands of years and long before confirmatory biochemistry proved them correct), asserts that no two patients are alike.

different food and chemical sensitivities triggering their symptoms. The Orientals thousands of years ago recognized that no two patients were the same regardless of whether or not they had the same symptoms. We all have different heredity, disposition, mental and spiritual make-up, as well as nutritional state, intolerance, and biochemistry.

4. **Masking**. Medicine must think a headache is a codeine deficiency. Providing a serious treatable cause has been ruled out, we are then trained to merely mask, or cover up, the symptom, but our bodies are already capable of masking or adapting by themselves. That's the very reason most people need to do the rare food diet to find hidden food allergies. They can have arthritis for years caused by beef and tomatoes and not see a direct correlation until they unmask or unadapt by fasting 5-50 days and then have the food again. Then, it hits them like a ton of bricks because the adapting enzymes were fooled into thinking that they were no longer needed (unmasking).

But what is the price we pay for this wonderful adaptive (masking) biochemistry so we can seemingly tolerate things that the body doesn't like? **Chronic illness** is the answer. The short term trade off for tolerance is long term insidious disease that builds for sometimes ten to twenty years before we know it's there. When it reaches a specific recognizable stage, then medicine steps in and diagnoses arthritis, diabetes, allergies, hypertension, or cancer.

But macrobiotics can diagnose your problem long before. And what strange terms they use—like you have hardness in your liver. What does this mean? You've eaten too many yin

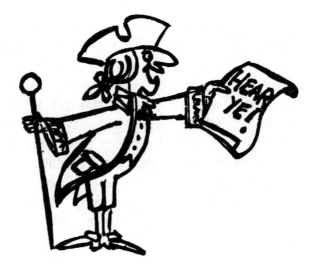

As dogmatic as medicine has become, it has been superseded by insurance companies which people have allowed to dictate:

What illnesses they can have, how long they can have them, which doctors can treat them, and which treatments they can have.

Only people, not doctors, can change all that.

items like tomatoes, sugar, alcohol, medicines, and caused expansion, or swelling, of an organ that was vulnerable. It lost its elasticity and became boggy. Then you continued excesses of yang foods, as well, such as beef and salts and caused a buildup of mucus and fats so that the flow of energy was impeded, or blocked; then the organ became tight and you felt fatigued and stressed (uptight). This stagnated area became a perfect breeding ground for infection and degeneration.

Add to that the acid diet (high in meat and sugars) and synthetic vitamin D2 that is added to milk and other foods; this combination fosters calcifications that are seen in arteriosclerosis, cancers, and many other degenerative phenomena. A high acid diet draws minerals like calcium out of tissues where they belong (jawbone) and deposits them in damaged areas (vessel walls). Synthetic vitamin D2 is an unnatural product that also breaks the rules of body homeostasis or balance. In other words, it is very deleterious to the feedback mechanism so that it actually enhances calcification in weakened areas. Once we have a hardened, calcified, weakened organ, we have the seemingly impossible task before us of dissolving this hardness and restoring balance. Do you think that there is a pill in the world that can do this? But correct body pH can.

Darned if this age old method of diagnosis doesn't scoop "modern medicine" with its fancy blood tests and x-rays. Plus, this age old form of medicine fosters healing in a way that is far more effective and healthier and on a a more meaningful level, as well. No doctor has the power to heal you; but **YOU** do.

5. **Total Load**. Medicine thinks a threshold is a level of

something that all people tolerate, and that it is a stationary value; in reality, it is neither of these. That's why some physicians get crazy when we tell them we're reacting to the new carpet glue, while the rest of the office doesn't even notice it. Plus they really question our sanity when our reactions are not consistent: we react one day but not the next, or have a headache one week and nausea the following. They are totally unaware of the detoxication biochemistry, when in truth when the detoxication system is stressed the maximum, a seemingly insignificant exposure can be intolerable and the symptoms can fluctuate daily depending upon the total load to a system at any moment.

And don't forget we also have a total mental load, as well. We all carry mental trash from years ago right up to two seconds ago that colors our reactions. Isn't it time to do some mental housekeeping as well? Start by working on forgiveness—of yourself first, then others.

Macrobiotics recognizes both the mental and physical total load. It recommends cottons, clean air, and healthy thoughts. The reason it recommends such seeming inconsistencies like natural gas is because of the electromagnetic fields produced by electric appliances. These can interfere with the body's own electromagnetic fields and detract from health. The problem is with us. We have gone so far down the tubes that we no longer tolerate gas; but people increase their tolerances to it as they improve through macrobiotics. At this point, because some of us may never be truly healthy until we get out of gas to allow healing, I cannot recommend that we use gas. I am not inclined to ever use it again, even though I tolerate exposures that I couldn't in the past. I'm not sure how far we can push our 21st century bodies.

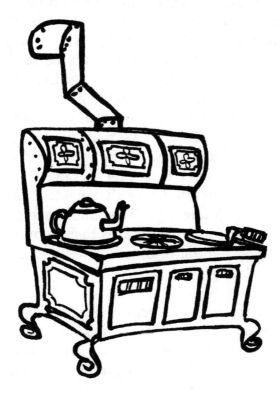

Nothing is perfect, including macrobiotics. Sure it would be wonderful if we could cook with wood or modern gas, but many of us have been so damaged by 21st century chemicals that we're intolerant of them. Avoid microwaves, as well, for they produce more of a disruption of life force in foods than the electromagnetic fields of electricity.

6. Likewise, **bipolarity** is unrecognized by medicine while it is a fundamental guiding principal established by environmental medicine.   When at first bodies are overburdened with a foreign chemical or wrong food, the adaptive mechanisms come to the fore (masking). People feel good and many (as I was) are in a stimulatory phase where they are really hyped up with energy.   As the detoxication and coping mechanisms become exhausted, end organ failure starts and they slip into the depressed phase, never dreaming that the things that made them feel so great could ever be the cause of such intolerable symptoms now. Hence, they set off on wild goose chases looking for everything and anything except the real causes that were right under their noses. And you can see how the initial stimulatory phase that made them feel good could be quite addicting. They unknowingly crave the very thing that eventually makes them worse. This leads to a downward spiral of obesity and/or other worsening and accumulating symptoms.

For example, Kate craves ice cream. She feels great when she has it. Eventually she has ten unwanted pounds, chronic tiredness and congestion. She doesn't find this out, however until she avoids all milk and sugar for one week and then reintroduces it.

7. Always remember that **the pendulum swings**. What this means is that **balance is not a static or stagnant** condition as "modern medicine" would have you believe. Remember when we were correcting nutrient deficiencies? At first we had to start with alarmingly high levels of nutrients to correct severe deficiencies that were present. Within a month or so, however, after the correction had been monitored, we then had to make a drastic change in

your nutrients and switch you from a corrective to a maintenance level. If you had been low in zinc, we would have eventually knocked the bottom right out of your copper, molybdenum, manganese, or magnesium, or maybe all of them.

The same thing happens with people who think they have the Candida syndrome. They start out on a sugar-free, ferment-free diet and feel wonderful for a month or two, but eventually they don't feel so hot anymore because they're having too much meat in proportion and have created a different type of imbalance. The same thing will happen with macrobiotics. You will start out on a more strict diet, but if you stay on this, with time you would not feel as well. You will need more variety and fewer restrictions, and you will need to balance your diet periodically with seasons and your body's demands.

At this stage, you may be asking yourself "What if I fail at macrobiotics?" If you've read through all of the recommended materials, and you have given it a fair shot for three to six months, I don't think you could ever be a loser. Even if you should not choose to follow the macrobiotic way, I think that through your exposure to it, you will have become irrevocably changed for the better. I don't think a week will go by in your life when you won't think of having some fresh greens to balance yourself out, and you will be more cognizant of the need of increasing whole grains. I doubt you'll be able to go back to a lunch of a hamburger, French fries and a milkshake. You're too smart to ever fall for that again.

The same thing happened with many people who looked at the rare food diet. Even though they knew they had hidden

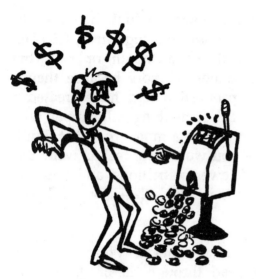

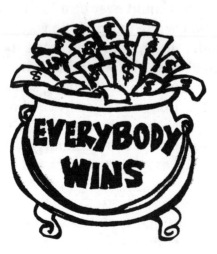

Life is a gamble, but there's no such thing as a loser if you are constantly educating yourself.

Even if macrobiotics isn't for you, you will continue to benefit after a trial, because of what you will have inevitably learned about yourself.

food sensitivities, they were content in ignoring their food sensitivities and being 50%-75% improved. They didn't want to go that extra mile and give themselves food injections or carefully balance their diets so that they could attain further improvement. Nevertheless, they sustained a permanent marked change in the way that they ate. Once you experience a more healthful diet, you are forever changed. You find yourself holding off on wheat for a day or two if you had been overdoing and not feeling up to par. For you have learned to listen to your body, and after all, a sloppy rotation is far better than none at all. As opposed to before when you were at the mercy of the food industry and their artificial flavor biochemists, you can't help but eat more thoughtfully.

Over the years, I have encountered many people that I hadn't seen for years and I anxiously asked how they were coping with their symptoms since they had left the program and what was happening in their lives. The majority of them told me that they had learned so much about foods and chemicals that they were able to handle their symptoms now without injections. Granted, they weren't at 100%, but they were doing so much better than they ever had before, that they were content with this level of wellness and optimistic that they could improve it with further environmental and dietary controls.

Remember, we only ever have two possibilities in medicine, and that is to medicate or educate. When I see these people, I know we were successful in educating them, because they are off all medications and they are masters of their own destinies.

Three more caveats deserve mentioning at this juncture:

1. Sometimes people worry that once they start macrobiotics, they will be stuck on it the rest of their lives. Not true. When you get truly healthy, you will find you can eat anything, once in a while. For example, many of us can go out with friends and have steak, wine, desserts, etc. with no ill effects. You learn your individual limits, which change with time.

2. Some worry about the severity of the discharge and whether it will interfere with work. But in the book (same publisher) **WELLNESS AGAINST ALL ODDS** is a detoxification procedure that can dramatically shorten the course.

3. Also in that book is the carnivore diet for people who eventually need meat, in order to reach maximal wellness. It is also the diet that people have successfully used to heal cancers when macro was not enough. So never give up hope, but keep expanding your horizons.

CHAPTER V

BACKGROUND & BALANCE

ARE YOU EATING OUT ON A LIMB?

So you see that medicine customarily re-labels symptoms and then finds a drug to extinguish these symptoms. If you complain of a headache, chronic diarrhea and pain, inability to concentrate and chronic postnasal drip, you might receive such labels as migraine, irritable bowel syndrome, depression and atopic rhinitis. These are medical terms for exactly what you've already told us. Then various chemical drugs are prescribed to mask or inhibit the symptoms. The underlying causes, however, are rarely looked for and even less rarely found. If you complain too loudly about too many symptoms or symptoms that defy diagnosis, then you're warned that you're approaching hypochondriasis and may find yourself seated on the psychiatrist's couch.

Medicine, a long time ago, gave the unspoken message that you can eat, drink and breathe whatever you want; that we have a pill for everything, and you have very little control over anything. Furthermore, if you are kept in the dark, this helps maintain medical mystique and dependency; hence fancy names for symptoms and drugs to maintain this distance and mystique.

But on the contrary, when the body breaks down and manifests a symptom, we should not lament and run for medications to mask the symptoms. Instead, we should rejoice, for our early warning system is beautifully operant. It tells us we are not in optimum balance and should do a good balance check to determine the cause before worse symptoms

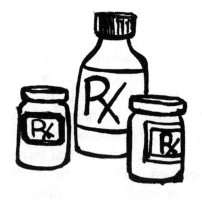

or

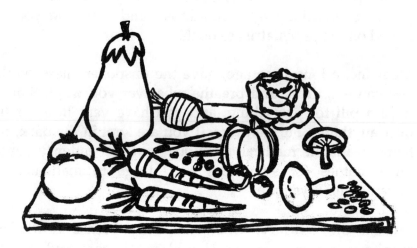

"Let your food be your medicine"
Hippocrates

appear.

Some people do not even have good early warning systems. They appear healthy for years, thoughtlessly eating whatever comes along, then suddenly they have a kidney stone or cancer. If you use all your income for vacation, you don't have any left for paying the rent. Likewise, if we eat for pure pleasure, without thought, we do not create a biochemical balance for optimal health and eventually there is a breakdown called illness.

The body has many buffer systems. These are chemical reactions that keep the body's pH, or acid and alkaline balance from going astray. If the body becomes too acid or too alkaline, coma and death result. If you suddenly down seven cola drinks, even though these are very acid, you don't die from acidosis. Why? Because your body has a marvelous chemical buffering system where it "robs Peter to pay Paul". Much like masking and adaptation, however, you pay the price. Chronic high acidity can deplete bones of calcium (it is one of the actual buffers) and deplete smooth muscles of magnesium. The pH or acid and alkaline balance is kept near 7.43 regardless of the abuse you subject your body to. However, when the system fails, such as in diabetes, a life threatening severe acidosis and coma occurs. You don't die from your seven colas because your body immediately brings this buffering system into play and alkalinizes the acid. The result is your body pH, or chemistry is kept in a very happy balance at all times. But if you unload this strain from the body so that it doesn't have to worry about balancing pH, what else can it do with this left-over energy, but start to heal? Healing is a phenomenon that the body does naturally by itself. But it only uses biochemical energy to heal after the functions of pH balance and detoxication have been sufficiently satisfied.

Americans in the 21st century, due to many socioeconomic trends, eat on the far ends or extremes of the balance scale. They eat mainly foods that are processed and contain pesticides, emulsifiers, preservatives, dyes, stabilizers and other chemicals in them. For many foods, often as much as one third of the nutrients have been removed during this processing. Also, tastes have changed in the last decade, as our modern food technology has developed. As a result, people eat way out on the end of the balance beam. They have very salty foods, they have very fatty foods, and they eat a great deal of meat. To balance all this, they eat sweets. Remember with the vitamin corrections, the more extreme a deficiency was, the more unbalanced or extreme the correction had to be. A craving is the body's way of telling you it's out of balance. The worse the craving, the worse or more extreme is the underlying imbalance. And cravings drive obesity, which is now at an unprecedented level.

Is it any wonder that the extremes of the American diet create extreme imbalances which manifest themselves as ferocious food cravings? Just as a severe imbalance in one nutrient necessitates a highly unbalanced correction, people eating this form of "normal" extreme American cuisine find themselves with very demanding cravings, or must have specific meals at very explicit times. When they're eating on the very ends of the balance beam or teeter totter, it's a very delicate and precise balance; the slightest upset in this balance can cause disagreeable symptoms. For example, many people know that if they don't get their coffee or their candy break or their evening high-ball on time, they're irritable or headachy or extremely nervous or depressed.

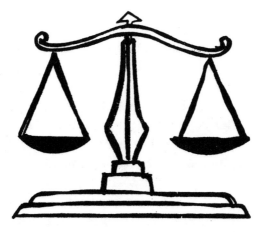

Your body is performing a constant balancing act. Salty meats (contractive) are balanced by gooey sweets (expansive), for example. Cravings result if you are deficient in nutrients and don't balance.

Or what about those who devour a huge meal with steaks (contractive) or roasts? No matter how full they are they need to have that dessert or alcohol (expansive) to balance them into a state of satiety.

However, if we bring our eating habits down nearer to the fulcrum, or the center of the teeter totter and eat a more balanced diet (one that is closer to nature and is more replete with the vitamins, minerals, amino acids and essential fatty acids and don't overload the system with unnecessarily high levels of fat, salt, sugar, and meats), a strange thing happens. Instead of the body working maximally all the time to balance or buffer itself, it's able to use this energy for healing.

Since foods vary in pH, all meals produce a resultant total stress on this buffering system. When the stress becomes too chronic, we get symptoms. For example, the diabetic prior to coma may have had a tough time healing cuts, may have gotten infected easily or had to have a root canal or had a bladder infection. Or he was frequently exhausted. But unfortunately nebulous symptoms can mistakenly be confused for hypochondriasis since they don't lend themselves to easy diagnosis. In essence, however, they represent the best opportunity to intervene before the condition worsens, for they are signs that one is headed for disaster.

So if you find yourself with a problem that just doesn't seem to be able to be totally cleared, it would certainly seem logical to consider investigating macrobiotics. After all, who needs to be eating out on a limb when the conserved biochemical energy can be funneled into healing?

Uncontrollable cravings, recalcitrant Candida and chronic

symptoms may all indicate that you're eating on the edge of disaster, forcing your body to perform an overly stressful balancing act everyday.

Who would dream of going to the doctor for food cravings? You'd be certain to be ridiculed or manipulated into feeling like a hypochondriac. Yet it's a true symptom of being "out on a limb" or too far from the fulcrum of balance. Take someone who loves a good steak and salty cheeses. In order to buffer, neutralize or balance this very contractive food, he will crave sweets, fruits, alcohol or feel extremely edgy and depressed and resort to medications. These are all very expansive. He keeps this balance going with little margin for error, always balancing his acid and alkali, and his yin and yang.

You can tell how precarious his balance is, by how embarrassingly bizarre his cravings are, or how urgent it becomes that he get his "fixes". The urgency stems from the fact that with the slightest upset in his balancing act, he begins to decompensate and feel awful. It's analogous to the withdrawal phase of an addict, for he can feel that desperate.

This balancing act requires a lot of biochemical energy and since we never get something for nothing, there is always a price to pay. The price is lessened adaptability to the environment, premature aging, and the onset of chronic symptoms. Excess strain on the chemistry over-utilizes pathways and their nutrients. This strain can come from environmental chemicals, balancing an overly acid diet and/or nutrient deficiencies from eating processed (nutrient-depleted) foods.

Take the persons who say they just can't get rid of their

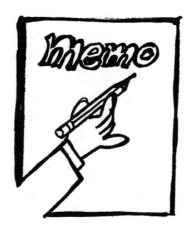

Remember, persistent Candida is not a disease. It is a
symptom that your body chemistry is out of balance. Once
you are healthy or balanced, you can't get Candida even if
you take antibiotics, and the cravings disappear.

chronic Candida. They feel they're walking on a tightrope because they must watch their ferments and sweets very carefully. We often find they do not possess a full compliment of nutrients when we check their blood levels of vitamins and minerals. We find they are grossly deficient in some of them even though they have been on seemingly good programs. Part of the reason (aside from food processing, depleted soils, and irradiation of foods, etc.) can be from the added biochemical stress of ambient chemicals. We're the first generation ever exposed to so many chemicals. All bets are off as to how the body will respond.

But bear in mind there's always a reason for persistent Candida. It should never last more than a year with treatment. If it does, there is still something missing. The biochemistry is not balanced. Some of them need injections to the newer molds that we researched and published in the **ANNALS OF ALLERGY**, (1982, 1983, and 1984) to keep their symptoms in check. More importantly, whatever the missing factor is that this required to reduce their total loads and restore balance, by not being able to totally get control of a symptom, suggests that they are pushing their buffering systems to the maximum.

The solution: do not eat so far out on a limb but closer to the fulcrum. This serves to lessen the over-worked buffering system and thereby allow the body to heal. This in turn initiates the reduction of other symptoms and lessens cravings and intolerances.

In other words, if every meal is carefully balanced to be in tune with the body, the extra energy needed for healing is suddenly available, since it is no longer needed for the chronic balancing act.

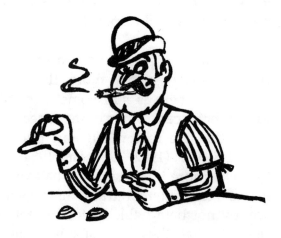

If you're not playing with a full deck, you will have persistent symptoms. You must have a full complement of nutrients, balanced meals, and have unloaded xenobiotics in order for your biochemistry to operate smoothly.

Macrobiotics provides such a diet. It is the perfect rare food or diagnostic diet (as described in our book, **THE E.I. SYNDROME, REVISED**), for it eliminates frequently ingested antigens such as milk, wheat, eggs, corn, citrus, chocolate, coffee, alcohol, beef, pork, chicken, etc. It eliminates foods on the ends of the balance scale. So what is left but foods in the middle like whole grains, steamed greens, beans, root and ground vegetables, and sea vegetables (seaweeds).

One way of eating back in the middle of the teeter totter or balance beam is through the macrobiotic approach. It attempts to keep the body in such perfect balance that it has energy to not only heal, but reach new states of wellness with improved emotional stability, optimism, and even increased metaphysical awareness.

At this juncture, you have noted the use of terms such as expansive and contractive. In general they tend to relate to yin and yang concepts of macrobiotics. Although neither is precise, they serve as tools for us to better comprehend what we are doing to ourselves with foods so that we can decide on an appropriate remedy. Acid and alkali do not relate to these, as you will learn later.

DRAWBACKS OF MACROBIOTICS

You might ask at this juncture if macrobiotics is so wonderful, why haven't you heard about it before and why isn't it more well known. The reasons are self evident.

The major drawback to macrobiotics is that it is different and we all resist change. It requires a total lifestyle change and much reading and studying. Another drawback is that it is not readily available in grocery stores and restaurants, and a third is that many people, regardless of how much they try, would find the taste of the food disagreeable. And it is not for everyone. We've seen people who had violent asthma attacks with every single grain. It simply does not work for everyone, nor does anything in medicine or life. Another drawback is that it can cause social isolation if you are not organized and in possession of a healthy sense of humor and self. And, until you get well, it requires frequent monitoring, nurturing and evaluation so that it can adapt to your needs as you progress toward wellness.

In the initial corrective or healing stages, it is restrictive of oils, nuts, fruits, meats, and other things for some people. But this is temporary as were the corrective stages of the nutritional programs.

The advantages, however, are that we have seen many problems improve that we were powerless to help. We also found that within a few short weeks many of the cravings disappeared and many incidental symptoms melted away, such as warts that had been present for years, or morning arthritic stiffness.

We've watched it melt away severe asthma, eczema, chemical sensitivity, the toxic brain syndrome (which includes everything from depression, exhaustion, inability to concentrate, spaciness, poor self-worth, undirected anger and hostility, dizziness, mood swings and much more), as well as non-healing injuries such as chronic low back pain, shoulder injury, and hip arthritis. We've seen people intolerant of non-phenol, non-glycerin injections and intolerant of any corrective vitamins become better. They cleared in spite of not being able to take injections, became more tolerant of chemicals, and even corrected their vitamin and mineral deficiencies. The seaweeds, for example, are rich in minerals. But any natural approach like macrobiotics takes longer than a correction with store bought nutrients.

As a physician, I have seen cures with macro that I never would have dreamed possible. Recall, Elaine Nussbaum, author of **RECOVERY,** tells how in her 30's in 1980 she developed cancer of the ovaries. After surgery it recurred and spread to lungs and liver. After irradiation and chemotherapy failed, it spread to the backbones and they collapsed. After a 2 year struggle with all that high tech medicine had to offer, she was bald, bed-ridden, encased in pain, full of cancer, 78 pounds and had pneumonia.

At that point, her doctors said she was so weak and so near death that they dared not even give her an antibiotic. She was given less than 3 weeks to live. At that lowest of low points, she went on the macrobiotic diet. I lecture with her biannually at the Kushi summer festival and when I meet up with her, she is often just coming in from jogging. She radiates health and vitality. She is now 15 years past her cancer.

Melissa Hatch is another lovely young woman who also in her 30's was given a death sentence as she had an inoperable brain tumor that was causing blindness. She went back to her neurosurgeon and he confirmed with brain scans that the tumor was totally gone. When I met with her last summer at Kushi's summer festival/conference, she was about 6 years past her deadly diagnosis. She was kind enough to send me a copy of all her x-rays and doctors' reports and her story is in the Kushi Newsletter, **ONE PEACEFUL WORLD.**

Do any of these cancer conquerors' physicians refer other patients to them if they are also on death row? No. And this is a great mystery when there are also scientific papers to prove that going on the macrobiotic diet more than triples cancer survival (Carter, et al, **J. AMER. COLL, NUTR.** 12:3, 205, 1993).

And this is in spite of volumes of papers, many published by the National Cancer Institute itself, showing that specific phyto-chemicals in particular macrobiotic foods (like sulforaphane in broccoli) actually stop the growth of cancers! They know some of the actual reasons and still it is ignored.

Macrobiotics doesn't make any money for drug companies, physicians, or hospitals. It takes control of health out of the physicians' hands and puts it in the hands of patients. The trained physician becomes your consultant and can direct you in your macrobiotic program and lead you to appropriate macrobiotic counselors and cooking instructors, and can monitor and guide your progress. But you are the one who determines whether the patient is compliant.

Initially, you avoid grocery stores and restaurants by opting for chemically less contaminated whole foods. It's actually less expensive to eat the macrobiotic way and, of course, far less expensive than organic rotated diets.

The pros and cons of eating macrobiotically are as varied as your imagination. For example, when friends invited us to dinner and nervously ask my husband what I could eat, he casually replied, "Have you mowed your lawn yet? She'll just graze for a while." Spring dandelions do provide a wealth of nutrients and can usually be found in organic form.

How long the macrobiotic way is needed is an individual decision. If one decides to stay on, there are problem areas that deserve monitoring, such as ruling out vitamin B12, zinc, fatty acid, folic acid, thiamine, and vitamin C deficiencies, or an excess of salt. We have seen abnormal levels of copper and thiamine, for example in newcomers. Although most people improve monthly by stages, some rare individuals require a couple of years to change.

Copy, fill out completely and bring with you the following questionnaire for your first diet consultation. Also copy and bring the list of food choices. But be sure you have read this entire book before your consultation. Let's see what your current balance looks like:

DIET QUESTIONNAIRE

Name_____

Date_____

Write out your four most typical breakfasts.

1. _____   _____
   _____   _____
   _____   _____
   _____   _____

2. _____   _____
   _____   _____
   _____   _____
   _____   _____

3. _____   _____
   _____   _____
   _____   _____
   _____   _____

4. _____   _____
   _____   _____
   _____   _____
   _____   _____

Do the same for lunch.

1. _____   _____
   _____   _____
   _____   _____
   _____   _____

2. _____   _____
   _____   _____
   _____   _____
   _____   _____

3. _____   _____
   _____   _____
   _____   _____
   _____   _____

4. _____   _____
   _____   _____
   _____   _____
   _____   _____

Do the same for dinner.

1. _____   _____
   _____   _____
   _____   _____
   _____   _____

2. _____   _____
   _____   _____
   _____   _____
   _____   _____

3. _____   _____
   _____   _____
   _____   _____
   _____   _____

4. _____   _____
   _____   _____
   _____   _____
   _____   _____

And your most common snacks or in between meal treats.

1._____

2._____

3._____

4._____

5._____

6._____

7._____

8._____

9._____

10._____

11._____

12._____

How long have you eaten this way? _____

What type of diet preceded this one and for how long?_____

Rate your meals by percentage. (The total percentage for each numbered category should add up to 100%) Grains (a whole grain is one that is still alive. You could sprout it in water and it would grow. Organic brown rice is a whole grain).

1. processed _____ whole _____ organic _____

Source:

2. grocery store _____ restaurant_____ health food store_____
   garden_____

3. cooked _____ raw _____

Food choices:

4. repetitious diet _____ random _____ rotated _____
   solo foods (mono-rotation) _____

Liquids consumed in a day (other than food):

5. over 6 cups _____ 3-6 cups _____ 0-2 cups _____

If you could feel like you want to tomorrow, list in order of preference the top symptoms you would like corrected, and the number of years each has been present.

	Symptom	# of years you have had it
1.		
2.		
3.		

4._____   _____

5._____   _____

6._____   _____

7._____   _____

8._____   _____

9._____   _____

10._____   _____

How many physicians have you consulted over the years for the sum duration of these symptoms? _____

Approximately how much money have you spent on medical bills for all of this? _____

Roughly what percent of this money was for:

Prescribed medicines	_____
Over-the-counter medicines	_____
Doctor visits	_____
Blood tests	_____
X-rays	_____
Surgery	_____
Hospitalizations	_____
Other	_____

How much productive time was lost from work or school due to these symptoms and consultation?_____

How many times do you urinate in a day? _____
defecate? _____
cough? _____
wheeze? _____
clear your throat of mucus? _____
sniffle and snort mucus? _____
hours sleep you need _____

Do you have headaches? _____ How often?* _____
nasal congestion? _____ _____
asthma/bronchitis? _____ _____
gas/bloating/indigestion? _____ _____
diarrhea/constipation? _____ _____
arthritis? _____ _____
fatigue? _____ _____
toxic brain? _____ _____
other (state) _____ _____

* Use Code:

     D = daily symptom
     W = weekly symptom
     M = symptom occurs at least once a month
     S = sporadic, less than monthly

Do you know of any problems you have ever had with your:
liver _____
gall bladder _____
pancreas _____
spleen _____
kidney _____
lungs _____
large intestine _____
small intestine _____
heart _____

circulation _____

glands _____

skin _____

bones _____

brain _____

Comments:

Questions:

Concerns:

Copy this questionnaire, fill it out and bring it with you for
your consultation with the doctor and/or macrobiotic nurse.

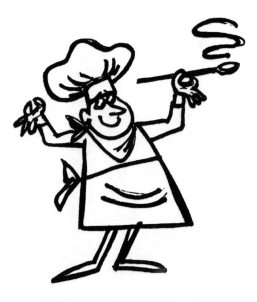

If you can't change your cooking and eating for 6 months, you're not ready to get well. You'd better explore why you need to hang on to your illness.

MY STORY

Even when this is all said and done, it was not enough for me until I saw the actual proof of the pudding with my own eyes. And the proof emerged slowly and sporadically. Several years ago a young attorney had colitis that surprised me in that we could not clear it with food injections. But he did clear with macrobiotics and was able to eventually graduate from macrobiotics and become even healthier. Then a couple of years later there were two young women who were intolerant of not only preservative-free injections, but all nutrients that we used in attempt to correct their deficiencies. Yes, they became sensitive to regular injections and had to have phenol-free; and then they became sensitive to those, and they needed phenol-free, glycerin-free. Then they became sensitive to even those. We looked at their many vitamin and mineral levels and found multiple deficiencies and every time we tried to correct them we found that they were alarmingly intolerant of the nutrients.

This provided us with an excellent opportunity to evaluate macrobiotics. After two years on macrobiotics, these two gals required no injections, fewer medications, and were healthier and happier than they had been in years. They were better able to tolerate natural gas and many chemicals that they were intolerant of in the past, and had indeed reached new levels of wellness. One became pregnant, having had several miscarriages in the past. A beautiful baby was the result. The other was able to work in a cancer hospice, because she was no longer restricted by her chemical sensitivities, and she, too delivered a beautiful baby.

Gradually, other people who were highly chemically sensitive started evaluating the macrobiotic process and started seeing some of their symptoms melt away. Having had nearly every diagnosis possible, I have always been the Guinea pig for every new endeavor in the office; it became evident that sooner or later I would evaluate the macrobiotic process.

However, I was at a stand still at that point, because my years of symptoms were infinitely clearer with ecologic management; intolerable migraines, chronic sinusitis, exhaustion and depression for no reason, chronic back pain for 15 years (after I had broken my back jumping a horse), asthma and extreme chemical sensitivity leading to the toxic brain syndrome and painful muscle spasms all were clearer.

I was healthier and stronger than I had been in many years and tolerating progressively more environments and foods all the time. In fact, that year I had lectured in four countries and a dozen U.S. cities, all the while maintaining a very busy solo practice, writing a 650 page book, a dozen health magazine articles, and teaching in advanced courses around the country for physicians learning environmental medicine.

Then, as fate would have it, I broke a tooth on a nut shell. I was deathly afraid to have any additional mercury in that tooth, since mercury had been one of the factors that had contributed to the downfall of my immune system years before; so I elected to just ignore it.

After more than a year, my dentist insisted that I make some sort of commitment and decide on how I was going to patch up that tooth. After researching the pros and cons, I found that all porcelain crowns and gold inlays required acrylic bonds or glues. These were deadly to me; they made me irrationally depressed and nearly suicidal; so I figured one

102

more little piece of mercury was probably the least of my worries. Besides I was so much healthier, I could probably take a high level of antioxidants and flush out the mercury, since we knew so much more at this point than ever before about how to biochemically detoxify ourselves.

So I let him put a mercury filling in. Three weeks later, after two hours of wind surfing, I started to develop a slight pain in my right shoulder. I didn't think much of it. The next day my shoulder was extremely painful. I sloughed it off as not being as young as I thought I was and waited for the next day when I surprisingly had even more exquisite pain. This was so severe it forced me into a sling and to take potent drugs, which I had been very happy to finally have been off.

After a month of being in and out of a sling and five months of severe pain, I called a friend of mine in Chicago, who specializes in amalgam problems. "Tom, I'm only going to tell you two things; one, I had an injury to my right shoulder, but the pain was way out of proportion to what I actually physically did to the shoulder, and two, it hasn't gone away in five months.

He said, "Right shoulder? I'd look at your right lower posterior molar" and I said, "You've got it!" He had known exactly what tooth I had a mercury amalgam in because the shoulder was in the same meridian, or Chinese acupuncture line, as the tooth that had the amalgam. I didn't even tell him I had had any tooth problems or any fillings, but by knowing where these meridians go, he knew what tooth should be scrutinized as a hidden cause.

The meridians are separate from blood vessels, nerves or lymphatics. They are part of an energy and electrical system which can be manipulated via acupuncture needles to induce anesthesia for example; enough to enable a New York City reporter to have his appendix out while fully awake and sipping a cola. When poisonous metals like mercury interrupt these energy channels, disease can result in any area relating to the disturbed meridian.

At that point in time I became very nervous, because I thought I would have to have the tooth extracted or have the mercury replaced with gold and glues. And if I chose gold I would have a mouth containing mixed metals (other amalgams and the new gold) which are capable of setting up tiny currents and creating new problems. Then I remembered my macrobiotic wish that I could be a Guinea pig to work out some of the bugs of this additional approach for those who might need it.

So I swallowed my medical pride and went to a macrobiotic counselor who told me many strange things and did diagnostic things that were very foreign to me as a medically trained physician. She looked in my irises, she looked at my palms, she jumped on the floor and showed me some yoga exercises that I should do and then she began to tell me the ways that I should change my diet.

After I left her, I was highly confused, but equally determined. I went to the health store and bought all of the strange looking seaweeds, beans and grains and root vegetables that she had recommended. Fortunately, at the store they labeled the contents of the bags or I never would have even known what they were when I had returned home. Some of the things were disgusting looking; 90% of them I had no idea what they even were or how much I should buy or what to do with them. The people in the store, however, were very helpful. At home, I called a friend who was well-versed in macrobiotics and she came over and helped me cook my first meal.

Some of the foods tasted wretched, but I ate them because of my commitment. There was a tea that was made out of fuzzy seaweed that tasted like dead fish had been rolled in it. That was to help kill my presumed intestinal parasites. There was another tea that looked like it was made out of orange red flower petals and that was to calm me down when I got witchy and irritable (who me?). Some of the seaweeds smelled like low tide at the harbor. And while I was cooking them, eating them was furthest from my mind.

I spent the next two days, (fortunately it was the weekend) reading and shopping. I couldn't believe how much I had to learn and at the same time I was constantly thinking how impossible this would have been for anyone else. Later that Sunday afternoon my friend took me to a local co-op and there I met other people who were also happy, friendly, and eager to help me. I also noticed they were very at peace with themselves, and with their approach to living. I was impressed by their willingness to give and share.

Within the first three weeks I began to like the foods and to get into a pattern so that I would be cooking up a big pot of grains or beans everyday to keep my supplies going. Several times daily I had to refer to my notes to make sure I had the right percentage of grains, greens, beans, seeds, roots, seaweeds and then all the special little teas, mushrooms and condiments. I was trying to learn some yoga exercises and skin brushing and trying to have positive and happy thoughts, while reading a voluminous amount of macrobiotic books on philosophy, theory and food preparation.

After three weeks I could raise my arm over my shoulder and swim overhand for the first time in 5 1/2 months. I felt so strange not to have that constant pain night and day. When something is with you 5 1/2 months and then is suddenly gone you feel naked, as though you've forgotten something. Also, I felt demonstratively calmer and more at peace. I didn't fly off the handle as easily and didn't have as much anger. When someone made an error, I didn't fly into a name- calling rage, insulting their ancestry. Instead I even floored myself by asking "Let me help you find where things went wrong and how we can prevent it from happening again." It was as though I had matured during those short weeks.

My chronic stomach problems that I had had the last couple of months totally went away and I had the most perfectly regular bowel habits I had ever had in my life, in spite of Candida programs and many food plans. I lost the morning stiffness that I had been having the last five years and there were other symptoms (like warts disappearing) that were definitely improved. These may seem insignificant but they are important indicators of the integrity of the immune system. Most of all I just felt so wonderful and happy and at peace.

Months later I went to my first dinner lecture at the local (macrobiotic) East/West Center. I sat down next to a cute elderly man and casually asked how he came to be eating macrobiotically. It turned out he was in his eighties (but looked younger and very vibrant) and had been told by a prominent local oncologist (cancer specialist) several years ago that he had only a few months to live due to spread of his deadly, malignant melanoma. He is totally clear of cancer today. His doctor considers it a miracle and does not refer other patients.

At this point in time, we're eagerly searching ways to make macrobiotics more palatable and easier to attain for other people, especially those interested in maximum wellness. But due to the tremendous individual biochemistry that abounds there is much personal tailoring that needs to be done for some to benefit from it. And macrobiotics itself is undergoing modifications in its philosophy, as its proponents realize you can't cram an Eastern philosophy down Western throats without modification and improving flexibility. As with any discipline there are the rigid, inflexible proponents, and then on the other side of the coin there are those who recognize the need for adaptation. At the same time, we must remember that macrobiotics extends far beyond just being a mere diet. It is a cosmic discipline extending to all relationships of a being. While this extensive an involvement many not be necessary for everyone, it surely will be for many. In fact for many, they thought the philosophy and lifestyle changes were more important to their wellness than the food!

Learning to eat the macrobiotic way is not as difficult an endeavor as it seems at first. At first it definitely appears utterly impossible and overwhelming. But in the first two months, not only was I strict, but I took my meals to Christmas parties, other people's homes for dinner and I even packed up all my foods and took them on a three week vacation to a Caribbean island where I cooked and ate strictly macrobiotic. This was a particular chore since the island did not even have many "normal" foods, much less any macrobiotic foods. But as we know, adversity is just an invitation to grow. And this served to help me get organized a lot more quickly. And it shows that we are always capable of a great deal more than we had ever imagined, and that excuses are only used by those not motivated to succeed.

Also, at the same time, I cooked double because my husband and people that we would entertain did not care for macrobiotic foods (especially at the level of cooking expertise that I had). So I made regular food for them. I was on a therapeutic or healing program, so I had restrictions and special foods that they wouldn't necessarily need to have, had they chosen to eat in the macrobiotic way, anyway.

It must be borne in mind that when people are healing, however, they usually will need guidance. The more severe the illness, the more important is the expertise of their consultant and the monitoring of their needs to change as the pendulum swings. Once someone has healed, the range of foods becomes much wider. By then they will also have gained more wisdom in terms of listening to the body and interpreting its dietary needs.

Someone who has a severe illness, however, should not even think about going on a macrobiotic plan, unless he can commit himself to having no meats, wheat, sugars, processed foods, and oils for six to twelve months. Macrobiotics is a slow way to health, as with anything that is worthwhile, it takes longer. It often takes a year or more for people to heal, depending upon the severity of their illnesses. But it has healed the impossible, where all else has failed. And people reach a more profound level of wellness than they have ever experienced before.

MACRO AND DETOX

There are many phenomena about macrobiotics that have fascinated me. One area that I have been very interested in the last few years is that of detoxification. As you know many of the people that we see with environmental illness have severe health problems because they have years of antibiotics, prescribed medications, illegal drugs, pesticides and chemicals that they have worked with stored in their body tissues.

These stored chemicals have damaged the biochemistry somehow so that environmental illness became manifest. Some people have fasted, others have done colonic therapies, others have gone to detoxification programs where they sweat intensely in saunas for several weeks at a time under medical supervision to get rid of these drugs and chemicals. All have had to do extensive environmental controls (as described in **THE E.I. SYNDROME, REVISED**).

It turns out that macrobiotics is also a way to detoxify and as I see it, it seems that it's a more beneficial and safer way to do it. We have seen people with the other methods develop severe nutritional deficiencies that required careful correction. But on the contrary, many people on macrobiotics have not developed nutritional deficiencies and we have watched them improve prior nutritional deficiencies without any vitamins or minerals. My vitamin and mineral levels after four months of macrobiotics were better than they had even been in the preceding years when I sometimes had to be on a couple hundred dollars worth of supplements a month. One reason is that the seaweeds are very rich in minerals. And some of these minerals are also good at displacing heavy metals like mercury and aluminum.

The detoxification stages, discharges, or healing crisis as they are called by people working in macrobiotics are an interesting phenomenon. What the macrobiotic people tell us is happening is that old diseased tissues are breaking down and old drugs, chemicals, mucous and bad accumulations are being expelled by the body. Therefore, severe symptoms will occur as these things come from the tissues into the bloodstream on their way out through the lungs, gastrointestinal tract, urine or skin.

These crises may happen 0-3 times and are preceded by feeling great. For example, a person may have a discharge or healing crisis with severe aching and recurrence of old symptoms like asthma. He may have mucous from the bowel, nose, or chest. And after several days or weeks of symptoms, he will clear and feel as though he has reached a new level of wellness. (Never fear, the duration and severity of a discharge can be dramatically reduced by the special detox procedure in **WELLNESS AGAINST ALL ODDS.**)

In a few more months, another discharge may occur and so on. During these times the consultant is particularly useful in being able to advise what steps should be taken to minimize the symptoms and maximize the process. Sometimes the process may be too much for the person at that point in time and they can turn it off and wait for a better opportunity. People have detoxed preservatives from old injection sites, old drugs (the odor will appear on their skin or breath, or they will create an oil slick in the bathtub or on clothes). My baby sister had an ovarian cyst. She elected macrobiotics instead of surgery. In a few days the area under her compresses turned black. The cyst was declared gone by the gynecologist. A surgeon friend of mine recalls a man with end-stage malignant melanoma. It is a deadly type of cancer and had viciously spread to his liver. There was no way he could live more than 3 months regardless of what was done. He accidentally met him four years later and was astounded. The man told him that since he had been given such a grim prognosis, he decided to go macro. In a few months he urinated black for a few days and after that the tumors and metastases disappeared.

RECOMMENDED READING

If you're contemplating the macrobiotic approach, you should start with this book, then **THE CURE IS IN THE KITCHEN**, which will show you the explicit strict phase program that cancer victims used. If that is too difficult at present or you are not sick enough and can afford to ease yourself into macro, then read **MACRO MELLOW**. Then **RECOVERY** and **RECALLED BY LIFE** would augment your understanding immensely. Following are several basic books for convincing and instructing.

A NATURAL APPROACH: ALLERGIES by Michio Kushi, plus the companion cookbook by Aveline Kushi, **COOKING FOR HEALTH: ALLERGIES** would make a good start for many. After a month or so then you would want to expand by selecting one of the following cookbooks and one of the books on philosophy.

CHANGING SEASONS, by Aveline Kushi and Wendy Esko, is a basic cookbook. Others include **MACROBIOTIC COOKING FOR EVERYONE,** by Edward and Wendy Esko, and **INTRODUCTION TO MACROBIOTIC COOKING** by Wendy Esko and Aveline Kushi. Then you would need some

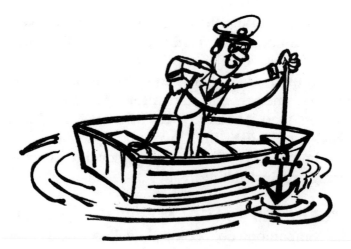

Let's weigh anchor and find out how some others have responded to the diet.

fundamental books on macrobiotics, such as **BASIC MACROBIOTICS,** by Herman Aihara, and **THE MACROBIOTIC WAY** (Michio Kushi).

If you want an inexpensive booklet that summarizes a great deal, read Michio and Aveline Kushi's **MACROBIOTIC DIETARY RECOMMENDATIONS.** As you get more advanced and curious, you'll be driven to **MACROBIOTIC HOME REMEDIES** (Michio Kushi), **THE BOOK OF MACROBIOTICS** (Michio Kushi), **HEALING OURSELVES** (Naboru Muramuto), **MACROBIOTICS AND HUMAN BEHAVIOR** (William Tara), **FOOD AND HEALING** (Anne Marie Colbin) and more.

Ms. Colbin has an excellent cookbook, **THE BOOK OF WHOLE MEALS,** which will enable you to make delicious, gourmet meals for the rest of the family, some of which will not be recognized as macrobiotic. Just remember, much of what is allowed there is temporarily off limits to you. But her two books make a great start for someone who needs a more gradual transition into macrobiotics.

You can order most of these from N.E.E.D.S., Geddes Plaza, Charles Ave., Syracuse, NY (1-800-634-1380) or Discount Natural Foods, Burnet Ave., Syracuse. But beware: many of these diet plans are for general maintenance macrobiotics, not corrective or specifically designed healing programs that will be mapped out for you after a consultation where it is determined what you will need. A maintenance program is for people who are no longer trying to heal any problems and can broaden their repertoires.

The only book to thoroughly spell out the strict phase macrobiotic diet that was used by cancer and E.I. victims to heal is **THE CURE IS IN THE KITCHEN**. This book will provide your foundation before your consultation.

There are no short cuts to macrobiotics, but fortunately for those in the Syracuse area there is an East/West Center which provides sporadic cooking classes, seminars, and a social milieu. One can purchase meals to take out and one can also go to dinner there. This organization provides a wealth of contacts to help you with your macrobiotic approach. As well, there are magazines, **Spectrum, One Peaceful World, Macromuse, Natural Health, Macro Chef,** and **Macrobiotics Today** which give many resources, such as books on macrobiotics and contacts in other cities.

Wouldn't it be nice if this approach became so commonplace that you could get a macrobiotic meal in a restaurant or on any airline? Indeed there already are some hotels and restaurants in the country that have macrobiotic breakfasts. When I lectured in Dallas at an international symposium, I called the local macrobiotic center and had great meals sent to my hotel. And it cost far less than the plastic fare at the hotel. Actually I have seen more macrobiotic meals around the world over the last decade. I suspect this is due to public demand. For there are progressively more people who have healed cardiac disease and cancers and must stay on the diet.

As people become more aware of the fact that their health lies totally within their power, I think the macrobiotic approach, as seemingly impossible as it might appear initially, will gain even more popularity. It can only do so as more people become hooked on their own wellness. A start could be by requiring their favorite restaurants to serve organic brown rice and steamed vegetables if they still want their business. For remember, restaurants want your business.

CHAPTER VI

CASE HISTORIES

P.J.'S PERSPECTIVE ON HEALING ALLERGIES THROUGH MACROBIOTICS

I experienced relatively good health as a child, and received honors for perfect attendance in my elementary and junior high school years. My family consumed meals from the four basic food groups. I especially loved cheese, fruit and ice cream. I became ill more frequently during high school, and my breathing problems were labeled "exercise-induced asthma".

While playing lacrosse in college, I developed tendonitis in both knees. The intense pain limited standing and walking. Despite many trials of anti-inflammatory medications, physical therapy treatments and cortisone injections, total healing took several years. In 1979, a bad case of mononucleosis interrupted my college studies for almost a year. I continued to have swollen glands and overwhelming fatigue, and was even more susceptible to illness.

In 1982, I happily acquired my first apartment in Syracuse, New York and worked in the Physical therapy department of a large nursing home. My health got dramatically worse, so I went for allergy testing and injections. I read several books and followed their advice to remove my feather pillow, stop using scented products, and eliminate some foods from my diet. Previously, my typical daily menu might have consisted of skim milk on cereal and orange juice for breakfast; mozzarella cheese on whole wheat crackers, peanuts, fruit and carrot sticks for lunch; tomato and meat sauce on noodles or white rice with a salad and Thousand Island dressing for dinner. I consumed small quantities of alcohol and pop, but had never smoked or drunk coffee. Gradually, as testing revealed allergic sensitivities, most of these foods were removed from my diet. Milk and beef were exceptions—they never seemed to cause any reactions.

My sinuses were always congested and infected. I sneezed frequently, and my sense of smell and taste had diminished. Polyps blocked my sinus cavities, inhibiting breathing, and had to be extracted several times. Each time, I vowed to do anything possible to avoid that horribly painful office surgery. I hated to rely on medications, but could not breathe through my nose without taking antihistamines and decongestants daily. I awoke 4-5 times a night to go to the bathroom and to get a drink of water for my parched mouth and throat. It's no wonder that I was always sluggish and tired in the morning! Despite these health problems, I enjoyed my job, had a fun social life and traveled often on weekends.

My future husband, Luke, had also experienced distressing allergy problems. He had suffered many earaches and infections during early childhood. Although his condition improved temporarily after a tonsillectomy when he was six, he became ill more frequently as he got older. Working on his family's dairy farm, he consumed lots of fresh milk, hearty meals of meat and potatoes, and delicious desserts. After college and a traumatic car accident, he returned to the farm as co-manager. Non-stop sneezing attacks while working in the barn left him exhausted—it seemed that he was allergic to the cows! He also experienced wheezing, incapacitating headaches and searing chest pains. Allergy injections and medications controlled the symptoms somewhat, but he continued to endure frequent colds, sinus infections, asthma, bronchitis and pneumonia. Desperate to feel better, Luke was forced to give up his chosen vocation and leave the farm. When he returned to college, some of the symptoms were alleviated. He continued to receive allergy injections for awhile, but often had bad reactions to them. Extensive tests could not detect the reasons behind his persistent headaches and chest pains.

For over a year after we were married, I took the pill for contraception. I didn't know at the time that it, like antibiotics, could upset the balance of bacteria in my system and contribute to yeast infections. I was being awakened every night by severe wheezing. Gasping for breath, I would sit up for about an hour until it subsided. This distress lasted a couple years. It was getting harder for me to work with my patients. The scents of their perfume, after-shave, powder, and cigarettes provoked sneezing and sinus headaches. I had to interrupt therapy sessions repeatedly to blow my nose.

I was referred to a conventional allergist for more testing. Desensitizing injections reduced the usual flare-up of symptoms during the spring pollen season, but overall, my condition had deteriorated. From experimenting with my diet, I knew that sugar and other refined foods caused many acute reactions. When I tried to convince this doctor that I felt that food sensitivities, especially sugar, caused my symptoms, he retorted, "You can't possibly be allergic to sugar— everyone eats it every day..." Surprised at his ignorance, I realized that I knew more about food allergies than this medical "expert"! What a waste of precious time and money...

The books I had been reading confirmed that sugar, cheese

and processed foods caused many health problems. By now, I could not smell or taste at all and was rapidly losing weight. Although I was accused of being anorexic, I was eating huge quantities of yogurt, fruit, fish, poultry, lean meats, potatoes, avocados and frozen vegetables. I still had strong cravings for sweets, pizza and other foods which I had eliminated from my diet. I felt deprived at most social events and celebrations where food and alcohol were emphasized.

Gradually, I realized that the air in churches, shopping malls, new buildings and my work place provoked nasal congestion, sneezing, wheezing, dizziness, inability to think clearly and sinus headaches. The fumes from our natural gas stove and heat, Christmas trees, and exhaust from vehicles were also implicated. We moved to an all-electric apartment and I stopped going to church and stores. It was hard to explain this to others, but Luke totally believed and empathized. He had been experiencing more headaches while working in a new office building, and was also bothered by scents and chemical fumes. In addition to sleeping at least ten hours at night, I took naps during my lunch hour and after work, but the fatigue persisted. Exasperated, I left my job to attend college part-time. I really felt alienated and cheated by my limitations.

In 1984, I went to see Dr. Sherry Rogers. At last, someone besides Luke believed that I actually experienced these symptoms. Better yet, she had confidence that she could treat me and reduce my use of medications. I underwent testing that revealed sensitivities to almost every pollen, dust, mold, hormone, chemical and food imaginable.

This syndrome of severe allergies was called "Environmental Illness" and I was classified a "universal reactor". Injections for pollens, dusts and molds eliminated the seasonal "hay fever". When hormones were neutralized, symptoms of PMS and endometriosis disappeared. Other improvements were noted when I switched from chlorinated tap water to bottled spring water. Unfortunately, I still reacted in various ways to almost everything I ate. Testing revealed that I was sensitive to almost seventy-five foods. Broccoli and rice were among the worst offenders. Daily food injections significantly raised my tolerance.

Luke accepted a new job which led us to Michigan. Once there, I discovered another enlightened medical practitioner, a dentist who was knowledgeable about the toxic effects of mercury on the immune system. He replaced all of my amalgams (silver fillings containing mercury) with plastic composites. My energy level and tolerance to foods improved immediately, and the nightly wheezing was less intense. Foolishly, I resumed eating some of the foods I had eliminated, and the recovery did not last very long.

In May 1986, my bout of pneumonia was followed by a week of immobilizing headaches. My balance and vision were distorted, one side of my face was numb, and high doses of narcotic pain killers couldn't subdue the torture. After one emergency room visit failed to detect the problem, I was admitted to another hospital. It was the worst night of my life. No tests were performed, no more pain killers were given, and I was not allowed to eat or drink anything. Unable to sleep, I begged every hour for something to relieve the mind-splitting pain. It was finally explained that the doctor feared that I had an aneurysm in my brain. Any medication would mask the symptoms and inhibit the diagnostic process. Intuitively, I knew that the problem was in my sinuses.

The next afternoon, CT scan results indicated "severely abnormal" conditions. I remained in the hospital for a week on I.V. antibiotics to treat the massive sinus infection. Further testing revealed that polyp growths densely packed all of my sinuses. Extensive surgery was required to remove the polyps, and my deviated septum was corrected. My nose hurt for months!

It had been an expensive and painful ordeal, but excision of the polyps restored my sense of smell and taste! At first, I splurged on a few treats (pizza and ice cream), but mainly favored large quantities of fresh fruit. We continued to eat lots of fish, lean beef, poultry, dairy foods, potatoes, granola and frozen vegetables. We often cooked in the microwave.

My general health deteriorated rapidly when I went to work in a new physical therapy office. My nose and sinuses became congested and my throat was so sore that I could barely talk by the end of the day. The thrill of smelling and tasting had only lasted two months. Within three months, I was back to the point where I could chew raw garlic cloves and not taste them at all. Poor health forced me to leave another job that I loved.

Luke drove me 8 1/2 hours to see Dr. Rogers. The exhaust fumes along the highway caused extreme lethargy and I had to use portable oxygen when we drove through highly polluted areas, such as Buffalo. I had recently discontinued my allergy injections because they made my arms sore. Testing determined that I was now sensitive to the preservatives. Fortunately, Dr Rogers was one of the few physicians in the country who had preservative-free extracts. I had everything retested. It was expensive, but the new pollen, dust, mold, yeast and food injections helped to reduce the total load on my system.

The following winter back in Michigan was frustrating for both of us. As usual, we were exasperated that illness was controlling our lives. When twelve different medications were powerless in fighting my bronchitis, I was forced to re-enter the hospital for more I.V. antibiotics and respiratory therapy treatments. The constant, deep wheezing returned a week later. Desperate for an answer, I returned to Dr. Rogers. She suspected a yeast infection in my lungs and put me on a systemic anti-fungal medicine. Despite the fact that I had been taking two to three grams of pure vitamin C daily, blood tests indicated deficiency. More supplements were prescribed.

Soon, the sneezing disappeared and I noticed a reduction in various sinus and digestive troubles. I tried repeatedly to eliminate or decrease the anti-fungal medication, but the horrible symptoms returned immediately. Frequent blood tests were required to make sure that my liver did not sustain any damage from the drug. I prayed that the tests would remain normal!

Meanwhile, after steadily going downhill himself, Luke finally consented to allergy testing. He also required the preservative-free extracts. Fortunately, they helped his headaches and sinus congestion almost immediately, but many other symptoms remained.

It was absolutely ridiculous! We had quit jobs, switched work places and apartments, eliminated alcohol and many foods, done environmental controls, endured extensive testing and injections, replaced amalgams, drunk only spring water, read many books, taken medication and supplements, and spent thousands of dollars, but still had not found the key to good health.

Dr. Rogers was the only physician who had ever encouraged us to constantly re-assess and re-educate ourselves about our medical problems. She had recommended numerous books over the past four years, but it was her suggestion to read **RECALLED BY LIFE** (by Dr. Anthony Sattilaro) that changed our lives! Inspired by this miraculous story of healing through macrobiotics, I reasoned that if this way of eating could dissolve his tumors, then possibly it would have an effect on my recurrent sinus polyps. I obtained **COOKING FOR HEALTH: ALLERGIES**, by Aveline Kushi. This book was invaluable in getting me started.

We had our first macrobiotic meal on November 11, 1987— Miso soup with carrots, daikon and sea vegetables, millet, and steamed Chinese cabbage. Luke stated that he would eat my new foods, but he didn't want to eliminate his favorite foods from his diet. Less than a week later, after observing my new enthusiasm for eating, he read **RECALLED BY LIFE**. It convinced him to wholeheartedly join "the experiment". I wasn't surprised. Generally open-minded, he was receptive to anything based on common sense, even if it wasn't "normal" according to others' standards.

After the first week, I realized that I no longer felt sluggish after eating supper. We went to see a macrobiotic counselor. By merely looking at my face, he could tell that I had previously eaten many diary products. In disbelief, we listened to his claim that by changing our eating habits we could heal our bodies and totally eliminate our allergies. It seemed impossible—until now we had only heard of ways to CONTROL allergic symptoms!

We felt hopeful as we outlined our long and short term goals. I had grown accustomed to the annoyances of frequently blowing my nose and not being able to smell and taste, but never having enough energy to do what I wanted was an endless frustration. My goals included being able to awake feeling refreshed after a reasonable amount of sleep, to have increased stamina and endurance, and a reduction in the amount of medicine and vitamins I was taking. In addition, I wanted to avoid having polyp surgery ever again.

We put our microwave in the storage closet, stopped frequenting the supermarket, and joined the local food co-op. We concentrated on chewing each mouthful of food thoroughly and stopped snacking within three hours of going to sleep. I read more, trying to figure out what the unusual words meant and how to prepare the new foods. It was astonishing—so many nutritious foods that we had never heard of! Surprisingly, I only reacted negatively to two of the staple foods: organic brown rice and azuki beans. They provoked sinus congestion, headaches, dizziness and depression. I cooked them for Luke and substituted other grains and beans for myself.

By Thanksgiving, I had naturally pink cheeks for the first time in years! I learned later that this was an indication that my lungs were functioning better. Another positive sign was that in only three weeks I had cut the dosage of my asthma medications in half. It was remarkable.

Although they thought our new beliefs in foods were unusual, my family was thrilled about my improved appearance and our optimistic attitudes. With the exception of the squash, we chose not to eat the traditional Thanksgiving dinner, and for a change, we didn't feel the

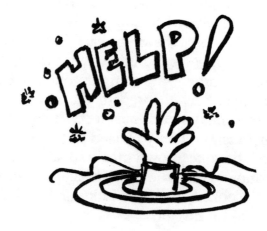

When a sound ecologic program is not enough, it makes sense to commit yourself to a trial of macrobiotics. But if Sattilaro's and Nussbaum's books don't convince you, nothing will.

usual after dinner overstuffed exhaustion!

We began looking forward to having our leftover Miso soup and whole grains for breakfast. This warm, satisfying meal provides a wonderful sustaining energy and is a perfect way to start each day. For a change, I had a big appetite and consumed frequent small meals. Never before had I enjoyed reading cookbooks and experimenting with different recipes. **My whole attitude toward food had changed—once blamed as the cause of many allergic reactions, it was now viewed as the most crucial factor in my healing process.**

One month after starting our experiment, we were convinced that this was the answer we had been searching for. We both felt more alert and energetic, we had clearer sinuses, fewer mood swings, more regular digestion and elimination, less flatulence, and better facial color. We had cut down considerably on vitamins and supplements, and I only required 1/4 of the usual medications to control the symptoms of my asthma and multi-focal yeast infection.

We were even more convinced of the worth of our new food choices when we survived the Christmas holidays without suffering from flu, colds, and infections that plagued almost everyone around us. It was becoming apparent that our tolerance had greatly improved! We could now experience stress, exhaustion, and environmental toxins without succumbing to the illness that usually resulted.

For the first couple months, we often felt hungry and unsatisfied soon after our meals. Our digestion proceeded faster since we weren't consuming the excess fat present in the Standard American Diet (S.A.D.—appropriately named). Gradually, our systems adapted to the switch from digesting mainly animal-quality foods to vegetable-quality foods. I no longer needed to eat constantly to feel satisfied, and we had lost our desire for meats and sweets. We had discovered some foods that we could eat in the car so traveling became easier.

After two months, I discovered that the breast cyst which had been unchanged for six years was getting smaller! I was amazed, but our macrobiotic counselor and Dr. Rogers were not—it was said that the cyst was a result of my previous dairy food consumption and would eventually disappear. The numerous moles on my face and body also indicated the storage of excess mucus from animal protein consumption. (It is a relief to not have to worry as much about them developing further.) Blood tests revealed no more vitamins deficiencies—my first normal results in four years!

By now, I could eat pressure-cooked, short-grain organic brown rice on a daily basis. I was delighted, since it had always given Luke a boost of energy. (He took it for lunch to work, with cooked vegetables or soup in a wide-mouth thermos.) Soon, I realized that I was able to accomplish more each day without getting tired, and I no longer needed frequent naps. In addition, I had noticed brief moments when I could smell.

I've experienced minor "symptoms of adjustment"—muscle and joint soreness—but no acute detoxification process. Luke discharged some excess mucus and toxins when he had cold-like symptoms for two weeks (without the usual fatigue and achiness often associated with a cold). In comparison with last year, our health this winter has improved dramatically. He missed an average of four sick days per month from work then, but has not missed a single day since our dietary changes!

After marveling at the way our lives have changed, Luke remarked, "Why did God give us the curiosity to seek the knowledge to improve our health? Maybe it's because we were meant to also guide others in their search for better health." I often shed tears of joy and amazement while READING **RECOVERY: FROM CANCER TO HEALTH THROUGH MACROBIOTICS,** by Elaine Nussbaum. I knew that every word of her inspiring story was true, because I had felt the power of this miraculous healing myself.

But how could we get others to believe that the food was responsible? Lend them the books! Having more information has helped our family and friends to better understand our reasons for following macrobiotics, and it has motivated some of them to institute some changes in the way they eat. (It is hard to resist the thought of feeling better, looking younger, and living longer!) After following some of the principles for two months, my mom discovered an unexpected benefit—the psoriasis that had covered her knees and elbows for thirty years had almost completely disappeared. In addition, substituting various whole grains and beans for poultry, meat, cheese, and pasta made it easier for her to lose weight quickly.

Now, four and a half months since our first macrobiotic meal, this way of eating seems "normal", and we can't imagine returning to the Standard American Diet. We no longer need the expensive medications, nasal sprays, vitamins or supplements. My endurance has improved considerably. Being tired at the end of a long day no longer means that I will be exhausted and sick the next day. At least, I feel refreshed when I awaken and don't have to be dragged out of bed. (I only feel groggy in the morning if I've eaten within several hours of my bedtime or splurged on excess fruit and snack foods.) We sleep soundly and require less sleep than before. Our sinuses are much clearer—it is wonderful to be able to breathe freely again. The postnasal drip that aggravated Luke constantly for twelve years is gone, and lately I have been able to smell briefly everyday. I expect to be able to taste food eventually, and feel assured that I'll never again have to undergo that horrendous polyp surgery! We are confident that my cyst and the dark circles under our eyes will totally disappear. We have increased the number of days between our allergy injections, and anticipate the day when we won't need them at all. We have enough energy to exercise almost daily, and I find that I can do more vigorous exercise in one day than I used to be able to do in a week.

I am much less chemically sensitive, and can better tolerate being in libraries, homes with gas heat, and some stores without the fear of having an acute reaction or "spacing-out". My talents and goals were inhibited by my health limitations for many years, but I am now looking forward to fulfilling my dreams of being successful in my custom wall stenciling business.

The exhilarating freedom of improved health has created other major changes in our outlook on life. We can consider having children (without the fear that they would be severely allergic or that we would be too sick to care for them). We can save money to buy a house now that the burden of excessive medical bills is gone. I feel a sense of reverence for the food, and gratitude to all who have helped to make our recovery possible. **I know that we were meant to be sick during the beginning of our adult lives, so that we might learn how to be well for the rest of our lives.**

Some people remain skeptical of our new way of eating. This is not surprising, since we had tried so many remedies in the past. Besides, the choice to heal oneself without conventional medical treatment is not well supported by our society or culture. It has become accepted for people to take medication daily to temporarily relieve their symptoms, and for children with chronic infections to end up on rounds of antibiotics or have to endure ear tubes or tonsillectomies. The probable underlying cause of the problems—what they are eating—is usually unknown or ignored, and new problems inevitably appear. For awhile, I thought I could eat anything as long as I took my medications. It was easier to do that than investigate and change the underlying causes. However, it was my experience that the symptoms only got worse as the denial continued. I am awed that something as simple as food could be the answer to many of the complex health problems that have perplexed conventional medical practitioners for years.

Most of us are afraid of the unknown and are threatened by new ideas. **It is easier to make excuses than to make changes!** Being committed to wellness means letting go of stubborn ideas, beliefs and excuses. It means opening up one's mind to new ideas, and accepting the responsibility for one's own illness and recovery. There is a valuable lesson to be learned: We each have the capacity to affect our own health and destiny. What you do with that power is up to you....

P.J. Tetreault
March, 1988

A note from P.J.'s doctor: P.J. is, as you can see, a multi-talented and resourceful survivor. She points out many essential ingredients to success:

1. A willingness to persist until the key to wellness is found.
2. Optimism,
3. love and respect of self and others,
4. a realization that in the quest for wellness, the degree of difficulty in the solution may be in direct proportion to how much you hurt, and
5. that food should be thought of as a friend and healer, not as the enemy we have perceived it to be in allergy.

An important warning is that many of us were not able to reduce or eliminate our allergy injections for months or years. All cases are individual. If you are not absolutely certain that you will remain on a macrobiotic program, it would be less costly and easier to extend the interval between injections to every 2-4 weeks for a year or two. Then in the event that you decide to discontinue macrobiotics, and/or that you still need your injections, you can merely tighten up the interval between them rather than completely retest.

Some people were told by macrobiotic counselors who underestimated the severity of their illnesses to discontinue their injections and they sustained life-threatening reactions because they were not ready.

REGISTERED NURSE, REPORTING

When I was an infant in the early 1940's, it was believed that newborns had an enlarged thymus gland and many of us were given radiation treatments to shrink our so called "enlarged gland". This was done to me. Consequently, the treatment took a toll on the proper development of my immune system.

Beginning in infancy, symptoms indicated I was allergic to dairy and wheat. I progressively added to these intolerances with new allergies. Some symptoms changed through the years, but I continued to deteriorate not realizing what was happening. Now I understand that repeated exposure to antigens (foreign substances) eventually depletes key components of a person's immune system. Aluminum accumulated in my body from cooking with aluminum pots, from deodorant, baking powder, and other products containing it. Nickel accumulated in me from excessive use of margarine, and copper from an unknown source.

Throughout my life, mornings were particularly difficult. I awoke tired, feeling like I had shoveled coal all night, and I lived for nap periods. Following naps, I yearned for sleep that night only to awaken the next morning as tired as I had been the previous day. This incredible fatigue was discussed with several doctors. I was told that I was fortunate to have my allergy symptoms manifested in fatigue rather than something worse such as asthma. "Which would you rather have to cope with, fatigue or asthma"? I left them feeling fortunate to have the fatigue.

My doctors recommended on numerous occasions I have surgery on my sinuses, even with this operation's low percentage of hope for reduction in infections. Fortunately, I refused.

I returned from every visit to my parents home with an incredible headache and joint pains. Arthritic tests would show a 4 plus positive for rheumatoid arthritis, but none of the anti-arthritic drugs relieved the pain. I later learned my mother sprayed her home daily with Lysol. In so doing, I was exposed to phenol. This spray, coupled with the exhaust fumes on the expressway added to the high degree of toxins affecting me.

Our dog infested our home with fleas. Three weeks following the pesticiding of our home I developed low grade fevers off and on throughout each day. At this point, I concluded I needed an allergist to help me. The doctor, Sherry Rogers, told me I was "environmentally ill" with severe allergies to inhalants, foods and chemicals. I was even allergic to the chlorine in tap water. With the aid of environmental controls, allergy shots and chemical filters (in my bedroom, office, and car), and thanks to my allergist I recovered a small percentage of health. I understood the only hope I had was to learn to control my environment in hopes of not becoming sicker than I was.

However, following one extended automobile trip with its exposures to the diesel fumes of expressways, I regressed and reacted to everything including allergy injections. The injections caused giant hives. It was a new symptom for me. This exasperating experience led me to seek alternative treatments.

One alternative I discovered was the macrobiotic diet. A nurse I knew, who also had been severely chemically sensitive, recommended it to me. This was a turning point. My health has been steadily improving since.

I visited a macrobiotic counselor who works with chemically sensitive individuals. She was my first experience with a holistic health approach. Using the art of visual diagnosis, like a Sherlock Holmes observation, she pinpointed many of my health problems. She observed that my kidneys were affected, based on dark coloration under my eyes, among other observations. Gall bladder and liver problems, hormones out of balance, intestines, etc. gave other indications of problems to the knowledgeable observer.

She gave me a written, "healing" diet to follow specifically designed for my condition. Seaweeds were included to help push heavy metals out of my body. Ferments and molds like mushrooms, wine, fruits, yeast containing foods, vinegar, etc. were excluded from my diet to decrease Candida. She recommended I rotate my foods as much as possible so as not to build intolerance to the new foods in my diet. Root vegetables were added to help balance the acid and alkaline content of my system. Beans and fish added protein. I started to take macrobiotic cooking classes to learn not only to cook the whole grains, beans, seaweeds, etc., but also to learn to appreciate what each food's benefits would be in helping heal.

A chronically ill person must adhere to a rigid diet to enable the body to rid itself of toxins and become better balanced. This healing can take a good deal of time depending on the severity of the condition.

Initially, when I began the diet, I experienced a "honeymoon period" when many chronic symptoms disappeared. Fatigue, constipation, irritability and depression, to name a few, left for a time.

But fatigue returns if I ingest a food substance I'm still sensitive to. Within 20 minutes of having wheat I'm sound asleep for 2 to 4 hours and exhausted for the following 24 hours. However, an increased use of whole grains that I'm not sensitive to, has given me an energy level I never dreamed obtainable. Much to my delight, I find there are no dips and peaks in my energy during the day.

The diet completely eliminated chronic constipation of 30 years' duration. On medical advisement, I had been taking 2 vegetable laxatives a day, and worried about the consequence of laxative dependency.

My cooking is now done exclusively in cast iron and glass. My aluminum pots and pans have been discarded. Since starting the diet I no longer require the use of a deodorant. When the chemicals in my body are being excreted through my pores, I do have a metallic body odor for 3 to 4 weeks duration. I've kept a couple of sets of clothes aside for these "off weeks". Including miso in my diet is helping rid my body of heavy metals and thus decreasing chemical sensitivities. Decreasing these sensitivities has improved my memory, concentration, and comprehension. Poppy seeds are helping to purge nickel out of my body. Sulphur flower baths aid in pushing all the heavy metals out, as do seaweeds and ginseng root.

Working through the years as a registered nurse, I perceived my medical problems from my typical western training, which is, to treat the symptoms. Chronic sinusitis was treated frequently with decongestants and analgesics. That medication exposed me to phenol and corn, two ingredients that are in numerous products, foods and chemicals. For the same reason, infections were treated with antibiotics (often on a monthly basis from October through May) which caused an overgrowth of Candida. That, in time, caused irritability, psoriasis, vaginitis, blurred vision, and cracking skin with acute pain at the outer corner of each eye.

Miso, if started too early in the diet, will cause the Candida to proliferate. I waited for my counselor to advise me when to include miso in my diet. My Candida is nearly completely under control and I've completely cleared my psoriasis, blurred vision and other eye symptoms.

I've learned that many foods that may not be tolerated alone could be tolerated in combinations. Millet, cooked with squash, and barley with rice, are often tolerated in combination, if not alone. When ingested by themselves, I became extremely dizzy eating millet, and experienced muscle spasms having barley. After cooking these combinations for a period of time, my intolerance to them has reduced and I can now tolerate them individually.

I've been told there is extreme heightened sensitivity when the body is cleansing itself of toxins. Many old symptoms are experienced such as irritability and depression. An acute awareness of this fact helped me keep the irritability in proper perspective (at times...old patterns of behavior are hard to break). The depression has completely subsided except recently when a chemical overload brought it on again. I reversed it with the use of pressure points (acupressure), another health aid I had learned.

The macrobiotic diet is not a simple thing. Foods cause the

body to react in definite ways. While on vacation I couldn't eat my normal macrobiotic diet. I prepared whole grain rice to take with me for my meals and ate little else for 4 days. Being new to the diet and not knowing all the consequences, I hadn't realized that a full rice diet can bring on a major discharge of toxins. In those four days I developed sinusitis which took 6 months to bring under control. I've learned to treat sinus infections with ginger compresses, lotus root plasters and lotus root tea. It's a pleasure to have a treatment free of antibiotics and void of the subsequent Candida proliferation they produce.

Since becoming knowledgeable in the macrobiotic way, I've learned that moderation in all things leads to balance. I can choose to eat in balance, or out, and live with the consequences.

In my 9 months on the diet I have learned that what I eat can bring on old chronic symptoms, be they physical or mental. Macrobiotics taught me the role diet plays in effecting disease.

The diet alone is not the whole story. It takes an overall awareness of what works best for each individual and the effort to do it. I can't say enough for the power of positive thoughts and the belief that you can heal yourself. No one can do it for you. And medication is a questionable aid. I found a combination of advice from a number of holistic health professionals and extensive reading gave me the tools to decide what was best for healing me.

I began to understand that I had to reduce the bombardment of chemicals that I encountered daily. This saturation kept my sensitivities at such a high level my immune system didn't stand a chance of healing. I had to leave my job in a building that was full of toxins (for a chemically sensitive person). The toxins included fumes from paint, cleaning fluids, glue, hair sprays, perfumes, smoke, etc. My health started to improve significantly within two weeks of leaving the building. But on three return visits the severe symptoms recurred. It made me appreciate that I had made the right decision.

Rooms were continually being painted and the fumes circulated throughout the ventilating system into every room exposing everyone in the building. Often meetings would be held in rooms containing new carpeting. Out-gassing formaldehyde from the carpet, and phenol from the glue underneath, affected people to varying degrees. When meetings were held in the art room, we were exposed to paint supplies and plastic container, each out-gassing phenol. Meetings held near the smokers' lounge left us with a prevalent smoke odor. Pesticide laden smoke from the smoking room carried into the rest of the building through the open hallway doors and ventilating systems.

Even when I walked into an empty corridor, I was surprised to be overcome with lingering perfume odors from employees who had passed by earlier. I tried to control the pain and muscle spasms from these mysterious exposures through use of pressure points. But often the overload of toxins my body was encountering during the day was too great. I was left ill at the end of the day with acute muscle spasm pain, laryngitis, headache and nausea. These symptoms would clear after remaining 8 hours in my bedroom at home with my chemical filter. Seaweeds helped relieve me of chemical sensitivities and made me more tolerant of exposures to chemicals. I'm now more tolerant of exposures to chemicals, and when overloaded, clear faster of the symptoms they produce in me.

Another source of almost daily attack came from my neighbor's laundry. Whether clothes dried on the line or in a dryer, a heavy, perfumed odor was exhausted. The detergents used in the washing process and the fabric softeners all contained fragrances and often phenol. The normal wind direction from the west blows the phenol fumes directly toward our home. When the laundry is being dried, I must keep all windows closed, even on the warmest days, and cannot go outdoors to use my porch swing or tend to my gardening which I've always enjoyed. When one neighbor opens her front door, the chemical odor of the laundry soaps all but knocks me over. I wonder what hidden toll it's taking on that family's health since they will have breathed the phenol each day and night over a period of years?

I read that "the human body has an electromagnetic field that depends upon body energy being balanced". I became aware of energy imbalances and how to correct them when they occurred.

Acupuncture treatments helped me by dramatically reducing painful muscle spasms that were caused by exposure to chemicals and offending foods. I gained an understanding of the use of pressure points that the body has, to allow me to control many symptoms of imbalance. I experienced ear aches when my kidneys were cleansing of toxins. This pain was relieved every day by a combination of aids using pressure points, ginger compresses to the kidneys twice a day, and 2 drops of warm sesame oil to each ear washed out with warm bancha tea containing sea salt. A happy added benefit is that antibiotics were not used and thus no Candida developed.

Yoga and deep breathing exercises have become part of my daily routine. Yoga has completely eliminated my chronic insomnia. I'm now asleep in 10 to 20 minutes, sleep through the night, and thanks to the diet, awaken refreshed.

I've been told that meditation may be an integral part of the healing process and plan to implement this in the near future.

I discovered the discipline of macrobiotics extends beyond myself and relates to patterns of behavior and interactions within a family. I believe that my entire family will develop balance and harmony in their lives. Through an increased awareness of each other's feeling and thoughts, our psychological, as well as our physical beings are effected positively.

All this can seem overwhelming. It is a new approach to health. It consumes a considerable amount of time just to cook macrobiotically. My advice is to do as much as you can possibly do initially. Don't become frustrated because you're not able to do it all at once. Take each day to add as many new dimensions to your routine as you can.

In summary, macrobiotics has enabled me to develop a better understanding of how diet effects the way I feel physically and psychologically, to eat in balance, and in the process, to unload many chronic symptoms. It has also made me aware of other alternatives that are available. I now realize that my health will only continue to improve in the future with the use of this valuable approach.

The end result should be an understanding of how to bring

order, balance, and harmony to your life. No one can ask for more.

by K.M. Swatt, R.N. 5/30/88
With much support and help editing and arranging
from F. Swatt, A.I.A.

I would like to thank Kathryn for sharing her macrobiotic experience with us. She reminds us of several good points:

1. Lotus root is indeed good, especially for lung problems. The reason I hesitated in adding it was that it's difficult to find in a fresh form that is not moldy.
2. The reason for failure to improve in a chemically sensitive individual may be that he has not reduced his chemical load sufficiently. Just as you would not ask a person who is trying to heal a wound macrobiotically to rub dirt into it each day, we cannot expect a diet to bring about healing in a system constantly bombarded by chemicals. If one has to leave work, it's advisable to first get proof of chemical hypersensitivity through testing in the office. Medical-legal proof is necessary for any form of disability, and is sometimes very difficult to procure.
3. If one is interested in beginning to learn the type of physical diagnosis used by macrobiotic counselors, two sources are Mishio Kushi's **How to See Your Health: Book of Oriental Diagnosis** and **Natural Healing Through Macrobiotics**, also Muramoto's **Healing Ourselves**.

D.J. was a 26 year old female with severe asthma and eczema over nearly her entire body. She improved with an ecologic program but her problems were compliance and money. If I could have taken her home with me and fed her and made her get her injections on time, she would have remained clear (as she proved when she followed the program). But she would cheat on the diet and not show up for her injections for months, then appear in tears. I recommended she learn macrobiotics. She returned to the office clear and happy, and it cost her far less than allergy treatments.

C.T., a 30 year old law student, had colitis that responded only partially to food injections and diet, but was markedly clearer on macrobiotics. After three years he modified his diet to include western foods and has remained in good health.

H.G. was a universal reactor, losing weight and a prisoner of her home. Within the first six months of macrobiotics she lost many of her chemical sensitivities and could venture out without a mask, gained weight, and in general felt markedly better.

The case examples have mounted quickly as more people have evaluated macrobiotics. Some have made more rapid improvement by amalgam replacement. In general, most people who attempted macrobiotics were successful at improving their chemical tolerances.

The impieties of our macro movement was evident in many ways. For example, if you attended a HEAL (local E.I. support group) meeting before we wrote the macro books and began teaching it to doctors as another tool to help conquer chemical sensitivity, you would have witnessed a rather colorless group with no makeup, wearing second-hand out-gassed clothes, and several wearing masks.

Five years later, it was a group infinitely more attractive (but the same individuals) , and able to indulge in makeup, new clothes, and get rid of their masks. The difference is many did macro or even semi-macro and decreased their chemical sensitivity. If you are curious how this can happen, **TIRED OR TOXIC?** has over 33 biochemical explanations. And since that time, we have discovered over 2 dozen more (many more are in the monthly newsletter and subsequent books).

As of 1996, we now have 9 books. You will see that each one takes you to a new level of wellness and is full of techniques for healing the impossible that cannot be found anywhere else. For example, **WELLNESS AGAINST ALL ODDS** contains the program for people who cleared cancers and other "incurable" problems but who could not do macrobiotics. Some healed with the carnivore diet, while others needed juicing and live foods. And **DEPRESSION CURED AT LAST!** gives further techniques for people who appear to be stuck and cannot get completely well. It is the protocol for finding the causes and cures of most diseases. There are other books in the making to show additional modalities that have healed the most allergic people, those with undiagnosable problems, those with ostensibly incurable diagnoses, or more resistant cancer cases. It shows we should never give up. And interestingly, some of these techniques are incredibly inexpensive.

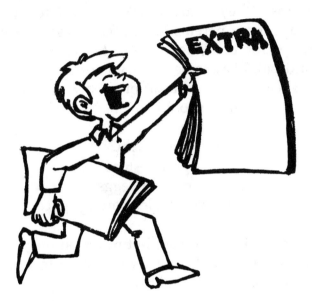

With all these successes, it's difficult refraining from cramming macrobiotics down everybody's throats. But nothing is perfect for everyone. T.A. had severe asthma. We had to test her to and treat her for her inhalants and food sensitivities. Every grain and grain substitute she tried with macrobiotics provoked severe asthma.

CHAPTER VII

GEARING UP FOR THE TRANSITION

THE BASIC FOUR FOOD GROUPS

You and I all know from third grade that there are four major food groups. They used to make me feel really guilty at 8 years of age if my parents hadn't fed me something from all four groups for breakfast. Being the oldest (of eventually eight children), I had to help everyone else get ready and was lucky if I had a piece of toast or a bowl of Cheerios. Here they were telling me I should have:

> dairy - milk
> grains - toast
> protein - eggs
> fruits/vegetables - orange juice

That might work on Sunday, but never on busy school days. As I grew up and got on my own, I found that the breakfast basic four could be quite delicious:

> dairy - ice cream
> grains - donuts or pizza
> protein - left over steak
> fruits/vegetables - chocolate

(you see chocolate comes from a bean, which makes it a vegetable, I figured).

Then as I got sicker, in my thirties, I tried to eat more healthfully, so the breakfast basic four looked something like this:

dairy - 2 glasses of raw milk
grain - English muffin
protein - 2 eggs with 4 strips of bacon
fruits/vegetables - bananas

Then when I got into my health food kick, it transformed to:

dairy - yogurt
grains - granola
protein - nuts
fruits/vegetables - apples

When I became terribly allergic, the basic four went out the window when rotation moved in. Breakfast might be four zucchinis one day and half a dozen shrimp the next.

MACROBIOTIC FOOD GROUPS

When I got started in macrobiotics, I was so overwhelmed by all the foods, I decided I had better devise a system to help me account for my newly found food groups. This is how I tally up each day:

grains, greens, and beans
seeds and weeds
roots and fruits

• Grains can be semi-rotated if necessary and can include (organic) brown rice, millet, or Hato barley. If intolerant, try teff, quinoa, oats, amaranth, buckwheat, or rye. Grains will change with the stage of healing and season. (If you have celiac disease, omit wheat, rye, oats, and barley and read **WELLNESS AGAINST ALL ODDS**.)

- **Greens** include collards, kale, mustard greens, scallions, parsley, watercress, Brussels sprouts, but later can be broadened to romaine, endive, Napa cabbage, bok choy, and more.

- **Beans** can be azuki (aduki), garbanzo (chickpea), lentil, and lima for starters.

- **Seeds** and nuts can include sesame, pumpkin, and almond.

- **Weeds** are the precious mineral-laden seaweeds; start with nori, arame, wakame, and hiziki.

- **Roots** include carrots, onions, radishes, parsnips, leeks, turnips, and the medicinal burdock and daikon.

- **Fruits** will only be "Fruits of the Earth" for beginners: squashes. This includes all hard winter squashes and pumpkins. Cauliflower is also acceptable. I also considered fruits to mean "treats" and use that word to remind me to add the miso or tamari to my dishes, as it was indeed a real treat to tolerate a ferment and something with a real taste after two months of G, G + B (grains, greens and beans). Other flavors (or "medicines", depending on your condition) could include grated ginger juice. Later a baked apple or pear or cherries, with steel cut oats once or twice a week may be allowed. More expansion and desserts appear as wellness occurs.

% VOLUME FOR EACH MEAL

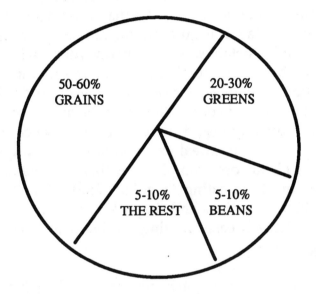

**TRY TO MAKE THE VOLUME OF EVERY MEAL
ABOUT 50% WHOLE GRAINS**

So you first learn to cook brown rice (very easy, directions later and in the other 2 macro books). Then you learn to make some beans. You can take 1 hour to do this or one month. The speed depends on your other life demands and on how sick you are. Once you master that, you only need to make them 2 or 3 times a week. Later you will see that it is also a perfect time to also make sea vegetables and gomashio, roasted sun flower seeds, etc. So that when you go to make your 3 meals a day, it is quite simple to merely prepare some fresh steamed vegetables to accompany your back-up basics. What could be easier? It takes 5-20 minutes to put together a meal and only 2-3 one-hour sessions a week to do the back-up cooking. And, of course, this could be just prior to dinner when you normally spend more time. In essence, once you learn it, it is not a big deal and you are not "always" in the kitchen" as I hear some complain. Eating macrobiotically can be just as quick as eating "regular" food. But it does not mean picking up a pizza and six-pack! That is not food. That is an accident/disease waiting to happen! The key is planning.

So for the first month, a quick meal can look like this:
- Spring water in saucepan, add diced carrots, onion, squash, and/or daikon. Steam a few minutes, add chopped kale, collards, scallions, watercress, Italian parsley, mustard greens and/or dandelion. Place cold cooked brown rice or barley and beans on top, cover and steam another couple minutes. DONE!

Now take inventory:
- Grains: yes, I choose organic brown rice today.
- Greens: yes, I'll have scallions and collards.
- Beans: yes, chickpeas.
- Seeds: no. So sprinkle gomashio (an easy recipe in most

of the cookbooks) over the rice or make sesame seed tea.
- Weeds: no. I almost forgot the seaweeds today, my wonderful source of minerals. Add crumpled toasted nori sheets or wakame. Or I could have cooked hiziki or arame with the root vegetables initially. Now where did we leave off?
- Roots: yes, turnips from my organic garden.
- Fruits: When tolerated, dissolve 1/2 tsp. chickpea miso in a small aliquot of the steaming water. Then add this back to the cooking pot and serve. Some days I serve the rice with scallions in half of a steamed acorn squash. And later you'll be able to make yourself real desserts.

Now check the proportions:

Item	Generally Recommended %	Possible Range
grains	50%	30-65%
greens	25%	20-50%
beans	10%	0-15%
seeds	5%	0-5%
(sea)weeds	5%	0-10%
roots	10%	0-10%
fruits	10%	0-5%

You see, you don't need all the food groups everyday. You don't need beans everyday, for example. And you certainly would not want all the choices in one group in one meal. For example, prepare brown rice for 1-3 days, then cook millet for variety for the next few days, then Hato barley. If you are particularly rushed one day, just make it 50-50, rice and veggies (greens, cauliflower, squashes or roots). If you happen to toss in some seaweed, all the better.

And when you get sophisticated, you can separate items into more elegant side dishes instead of making one casserole-type meal. For example, you could start with the roots and "fruits" in the form of carrots in miso soup. Then make another side dish of white baby lima beans in Kombu, another of brown rice with toasted sesame seeds (gomashio), and one of steamed kale. There you have a macrobiotic meal with 4 dishes.

Congratulations: You have mastered one of the most difficult transitions of going from an American fast food diet into a healthful whole grains and fresh vegetable macrobiotic diet. In a few weeks, you will be on your way to a new level of wellness. If it seems too extreme, you may be happier with a more gradual transition. One option is to merely reduce your portions of everything you normally eat by 50%. Make up the difference in brown rice and kale, 50-50. They will not taste great, however, because your taste buds are being bludgeoned by the extreme tastes of your regular foods.

THE TRANSITION: GO FOR IT

The transition to macrobiotics can be done in many ways. You could start by cutting out sweets and meats, the two most common extremes. So in order to have something to eat, you'd better slip in a whole, unbroken grain to every meal. So your first macrobiotic food will probably be organic brown rice. Try to work it up to 50% of each meal. Don't worry if you're not perfect - you're learning, so go easy on yourself. Next get some steamed greens into each meal and try for 25%.

Remember to chew very well. I used to bolt my food; one to three bites was usually max for me before I swallowed. But considering what I ate, it didn't require much chewing. When you eat whole grains, however, you should chew each mouthful until it is totally liquid. (1) It unloads your pancreas from unnecessary work, thereby helping your body heal hypoglycemia and other problems. (2) Saliva can actually change the food from acid to alkaline. (3) It increases and improves the amount of nutrients you get from the food.

Back to your transition, Shirley Gallinger's **MACRO MELLOW** has guided many (available through this publisher). Or you could read Colbin's, **THE BOOK OF WHOLE MEALS**. Both books not only have recipes but menus and preparation time schedules. Then just ease on into that transition. While phasing out sweets, meats, and dairy, phase in grains and greens. Hopefully from your E.I. experience you already are smart enough to be off processed foods.

Before macrobiotics I probably had beans and whole grains maybe once a year. I remember I made a barley soup once and had once cooked some brown rice just out of curiosity to see what the big deal was. Since neither one was as delicious (then!) as my sticky buns, I decided they took too long and were not worth the effort. So I left my beans to yearly picnics and decided to get my whole grains from oatmeal cookies!

Sadly, most of us have totally ignored whole grains, beans and many greens most of our lives. We actually had to learn how to cook brown rice, aduki and collards.

In the beginning you'll probably find it impossible to believe (as we all did) that your sweet craving can be controlled with sweet vegetables or balanced with sour (umeboshi). Or that your bitter craving (beer, coffee, cigarettes) will be controlled with bitter vegetables (endive, dandelion, escarole, chicory). But as you begin to get off the extremes of meats and sweets, and onto a more easily buffered whole grains and veggies diet, these extremes will no longer have as much appeal.

Your first cooking priority is to start with grains and beans. What I do now is cook both two or three times a week so I have them ready for a couple of days to add to meals.

A word about washing grains: I thought it was silly to wash grains and beans — after all you boil them! But by washing the grain you remove dust and dirt, fine stones (I've found some boulders!) that can break teeth and you remove the rodent feces. Most importantly, you wash off some mycotoxins that are toxins made by molds that are invisible, tasteless, and odorless, but capable of causing cancer.

So how does one go about starting on a macrobiotic program? Probably the first thing you need is commitment. Weigh the pros and cons critically to see if you really have the commitment. What's the worst thing that could happen with macrobiotics? First, there could be absolutely no benefit. Second, you may lose much weight. Third, you may lose your friends since you won't be eating meals at their houses, but that's easily remedied, since you can bring your own foods. Fourth, you will have to totally change your cooking, shopping and eating patterns and do a tremendous amount of reading, which will take time away from other activities. Fifth, if you don't go on a program appropriately with monitoring, you could make your symptoms worse and develop nutritional deficiencies. Sixth, you often have seaweed in your teeth.

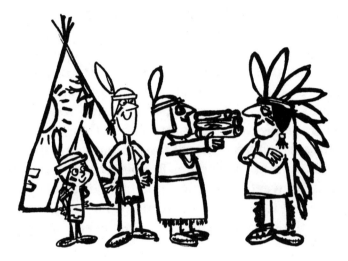

For starters, make a trade:
meats and sweets
for
grains and greens.

And what's the best that can happen on macrobiotics? Obviously, you have a strong chance of clearing conditions that have resisted many other therapies and been termed incurable. You may arrive at new levels of health that you never dreamed possible.

How do you begin such an insurmountable task as starting a macrobiotic program? First, go to the grocery store and buy some hard yellow or green winter squashes, such as acorn squashes, some large yellow onions, carrots, and scallions. Then go to an oriental market or health food store for a large fat root called daikon. Cut up a cup of each of these (squash, onion, carrot, daikon) into bite size pieces and add four cups of water to a pot and a pinch of salt and boil it for twenty minutes until the vegetables are soft. This is your "squash soup". In a pinch you can eat it for breakfast with precooked brown rice, or add the veggies to your casserole. Because it is composed of sweet vegetables, it helps the sweet cravings and hypoglycemia that many newcomers have. If they persist, you have mineral deficiencies we can correct.

Next, buy a pressure cooker and cook several cups of brown rice. Also, buy some greens at the grocery. Hard greens such as kale, collards, or mustard greens are preferable; also dandelion, parsley, watercress, or scallions can be used, as well as cauliflower, leeks, onion, parsnip, carrots, any hard winter pumpkins or squashes, Brussels sprouts, turnips and radishes. Napa cabbage or romaine lettuce would suffice if the other greens are not available. Also, purchase some assorted beans, such as chickpeas or garbanzo beans as well as aduki beans. All the beans, grains, and specialty items like sea vegetables and miso can all be purchased by mail through Mountain Ark Trading Company, Fayetteville, Arkansas 1-800-643-8905 and Goldmine Natural Food Company, San

Diego California, 1-800-475-FOOD, and Natur-Tyme West, Syracuse, New York 1-800-634-1380. Most of these places will carry items you need if you only ask. I actually prefer to order by mail since it saves me time, driving, and shopping. Also the items come labeled when you shop by mail, and in the beginning most people don't know hiziki from wakame.

Sometimes, people who live in isolated areas think that it makes eating macrobiotically impossible. That is not true. You merely order the grains, beans, seeds, condiments and seaweeds from catalogs. Then use your local grocer for whatever veggies (above and below ground) that you can get. If you are limited to cabbage, carrots, onions and hard squashes, that is not a problem.

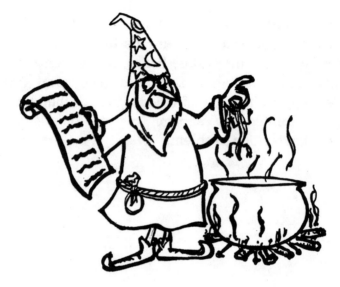

Some of the sights and smells will give you second thoughts,
but TRUST ME. Have I ever steered you wrong?

You can start out the first week rather simply. Put 1/2 cup of the squash soup liquid in a fry pan. Add some arame seaweed (which is an excellent source of minerals) to the veggie water and cook about two minutes. Then add the precooked rice just to re-heat it. You can add the precooked veggies here if any remain (or add new ones to the seaweed cooking cycle that preceded this since additional uncooked ones would require more cooking time). You can also cut up some of the kale or other greens and scallions and steam the whole thing in just two minutes. If more water is necessary, add it to this mixture. This can be eaten for breakfast, lunch, and dinner for the first couple of days or weeks until you start getting acclimated to the other foods and the recipes. There are many variations, and you'll need to progress beyond this within a month.

Until you get your bearings, you could exist on this a week or more (I did, for over three months, as a trial). It's quick and easy to organize. Two or three times a week cook your squash drink, grains, and beans. When mealtime comes, first prepare everyone else's regular food. In the last minutes, cook your roots (onion, daikon, burdock, etc.), and seaweed in the squash soup juice or water for 5 minutes, add the precooked grains and beans and the chopped greens for another 2 to 3 minutes of cooking and you're ready to eat. The grains are warmed in the time the greens are steamed. Take inventory to see if you have included grains, greens and beans, weeds and seeds, roots and fruits. Sprinkle gomashio over the rice and mix in miso (and/or some ginger juice) if you can tolerate it yet. Check your proportions and serve. Now if you can't manage that, you don't have a burning desire to get well; it's more like a flicker.

You will notice you are able to eat much larger amounts of

foods than you ever did before and that you will start dropping weight. This is fine, because fat contains the foreign chemicals or xenobiotics, which need to be detoxified. You can put back the weight later on with good, clean organic food.

You can use roasted barley tea as an in between drink, or once a week in the transition stage, some boiled almonds with the peels off. Simply squeeze them after they've been boiled for 10 minutes in water and they will pop out of their skins. Easy digestibility is an important factor and so is peace; each meal should be taken with a preliminary grace, expressing gratitude for the meal and good thoughts throughout the meal with very meticulous and thorough chewing. All foods and drinks must be well mixed with saliva to start breaking down the materials for proper digestion and assimilation. Most sick people have the leaky gut syndrome as described in **WELLNESS AGAINST ALL ODDS**, and these measures promote the healing of it.

In the evening you can add a half a cup or more of the beans, as well, to this mixture. You may be in a rush in the morning and choose to only have the squash soup or only the rice; then again you may have everything. You don't need beans at every meal or even every day. Substitute some vegetables like hard squash, cauliflower, or Brussels sprouts. You don't need greens at every meal. But these are good guidelines. Much depends on whether you are doing a **transitional diet** (just getting used to whole foods and less meat, sweets, and dairy), a **healing diet** (which is the most strict of all), or a fun and creative **maintenance diet** (which can be masked "American" fare by talented cooks). Whichever, don't immerse yourself in guilt. There is no absolute right or wrong and learning is a commendable process.

Eventually you want to aim for at least 30 to 50% of each day's food and preferably each meal to be a whole grain, such as rice, oat, millet, barley, etc. It is best to start with rice the first week until you are sure of what other foods you should be having. If you're allergic to rice, try millet, corn, rye, oats, barley. Then try amaranth, quinoa (pronounced keen'wah), or buckwheat, since they are out of the grass family. If not successful, be sure they were organic before resorting to tapioca or "non-grains" for a while. A consultation can provide further guidance, as can **THE CURE IS IN THE KITCHEN**.

At least 50% of the total diet should be vegetables. This includes greens, gourds (squashes) and root vegetables (turnips, carrots, onions, burdock, daikon), seaweeds, beans, nuts, and seeds as well as condiments and teas. Occasionally beer and sake are allowed after healing when a much broader diet is introduced. And some people really need red meat periodically after wellness has been attained. Nothing is cast in stone as evidenced by healthy specimens from all cultures. Many people need raw fruits and vegetables daily. There is much to be said for the life force which exists in living foods.

But if one is going to go on a program specifically for healing through macrobiotics, he should be resigned to the fact that most likely during the first six to twelve months he will not have any meats, sweets, processed foods, or fruits. If this type of commitment could not be made, I suggest the macrobiotic approach should not be considered.

There are other ways to deal with this, such as slowly introducing macrobiotic foods, but it appears that the cold turkey method is the best way to start to stomp out food cravings. Also, it's very difficult to appreciate the sweetness and goodness in many vegetables, such as carrots, turnips, onions and squashes when one is still eating honey, sugar, corn and cane sweeteners as well as artificial sweeteners. These strong sweeteners blunt the taste buds severely, or cause imbalances in the body chemistry, thereby maintaining cravings.

QUICK SUMMARY

1. Stop meats, sweets, dairy. (This assumes you are health oriented enough to already have been off processed foods including alcohol and coffee.)

2. Begin 50-50 whole grains and vegetables.

3. Further refine to grains, greens and beans, seeds and sea) weeds, roots and "fruits". Watch that proportions are accurate.

FOOD CHOICES
ORGANIZATION BEGINS WITH A LIST

Make copies of the following pages, right up to the Suggested Menu. Bring them to your consultation to check off what foods you can have. Then you have a ready made list to carry to the store for shopping as well.

In the meantime you will want to start making a list for your needs. From the grocery store you will need some **greens**:

scallions	dandelion greens
mustard greens	parsley

kale	watercress
rappi	cabbage
collard greens	Brussels sprouts

Grow alfalfa sprouts on your windowsill. Use cabbage or romaine if none of the above greens are available. We know these are not all available. Two or three from the list per week is fine. You do not need them all.

From the health food store or mail order catalogue, you will need a good supply of medium grain brown rice, and you may want to have some short grain, as well. These can be rotated with other grains to avoid further sensitization.

medium grain brown rice
millet
rye
Hato barley

If you don't tolerate any of the above, try:

corn	amaranth
quinoa	buckwheat
teff	oats

(Bulgar, spelt, and couscous are wheat derived and somewhat processed, so avoid them unless they are the only ones tolerated).

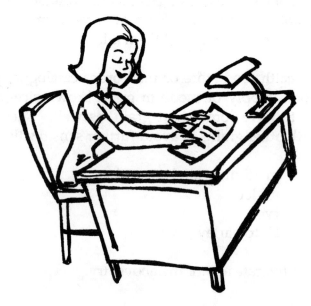

You'll need to organize your food needs by where you will purchase them. You don't have time to waste running all over the city looking for obscure items. You'll find you shop less at the grocer and more at the co-op or health food store. Share the trips with your buddy. It's so easy to make a list of your needs; you can also do it by mail, as I do.

Most of the vegetables can be obtained at the grocery except burdock, lotus and daikon, which are not always available, but Natural Discount Foods, Natur-Tyme West, Whole Earth Foods and the Oriental House often have some seasonal items.

Above Ground	Below Ground
cauliflower	carrots (+ tops)
hard winter squashes	onions (+tops)
cabbage	burdock root
Brussels sprouts	lotus root
leeks	turnips
	daikon (+tops)
	radish (+tops)
	parsnips (+tops)

Condiments:
Umeboshi (erroneously called "plums" everywhere, but Michio Kushi tells me they are really apricots. The term got lost in translation years ago, just as yin and yang got accidentally reversed, leading to much confusion. Anyway, umeboshi "plums" are very salty tasting but they can alkalinize you like alka-aid did for food and chemical reactions - see **THE E.I. SYNDROME, REVISED).**

wheat-free tamari   sage
chickpea miso   sea salt
shitake mushrooms (one a week only)
ginger root (for compresses, tea, or flavoring)
thyme
scallions
sesame seeds (to make your gomashio)
wakame (for seaweed powder)

Beans:

lentil	split pea	pinto	lima
azuki	chickpeas	navy	mung

Seaweeds:

nori	arame	kombu
wakame	hiziki	sea palm

Oils:

Occasional olive or unrefined sesame (oils are usually not used in healing phase. Just stick to steaming until a consultation.)

Teas:

bancha	safflower
roasted barley	roasted rice
sesame	spring water

Meat:

White fishes, including red snapper, halibut, shrimp, haddock, all with grated daikon/tamari (maximum twice a week in transition phase and wean to once every 2-4 weeks in healing phase, unless you need the calories and protein).

Sweets and snacks: (Use very sparingly for healing; use only if you must, maximum once a week)

> yinnie rice syrup (on hot cereal grain)
> cooked fruits (apple, pear, cherries)
> chestnuts (available in late fall)
> rice cakes with tahini and yinnie syrup
> boiled, peeled almonds
> roasted pumpkin seeds with tamari
> mugwort mochi with daikon/tamari

popcorn (air popped, no salt or butter)
sunflower seeds (roasted in fry pan or raw)

Cooking tools:
Aeterum pressure cooker
2 stainless steel sauce pans
2 stainless steel fry pans
1 good chef's knife
1 good paring knife
1 vegetable peeler
2 colanders, large and medium
1 bamboo tea strainer
1 hand grater
1 sushi mat
1 spatula
1 wooden spoon
1 suribachi with pestle
8 large glass storage jars for grains and seaweeds
8 medium size glass storage jars for beans and nuts
8 smaller size glass storage jars for teas, mushrooms and seeds
2 wide mouth thermoses for work and travel
1 or 2 covered, divided dishes for work and travel
1 small picnic cooler for work and travel

Obviously, you can't run out and get everything, but work into your needs. Also, you may discover many of these items at garage sales, for example.

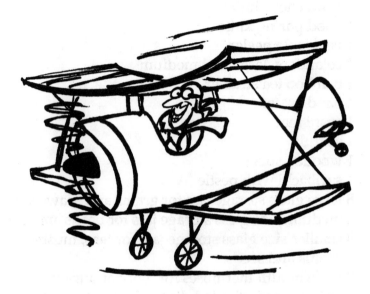

If it's a very long trip, order the vegetarian meals and pick at a dry salad and whatever else you can use. Bring along umeboshi-nori rolls and bottled water or bancha tea.

The following items may be allowed early, later on as a medicinal therapy, or not until you are better. You can **bring this list to your consultation** to check off things that you could be having. Do not have them initially until you have had a consultation, but instead limit your diet to the items on the previous pages only.

Grains
corn
wheat berries
(Essene bread)
noodles, udon
flour products

Beans
kidney
Nato
soy
tempeh
tofu

Sea Vegetables
agar-agar
dulse
Irish moss
mekabu
sea palm
kelp

Vegetables
broccoli
celery
cucumber
endive
escarole
green beans
peas
Jerusalem artichokes
kohlrabi
mushrooms
summer squashes

Fruits
apples
blueberries
cherries
grapes
melons
peaches
pears
plums
raisins
strawberries

Seeds
chestnuts
sunflower seeds

Teas
Corsican
dandelion
kombu
mu
nettle

Meats
clams
lobster
white fish (cod, flounder, halibut, sole, snapper)
shrimp

Pickles and sauerkraut
wash salt from sauerkraut

Sweets	**Oils**	**Other**
amazake	sesame	miso
apple juice	unrefined olive	shitake
barley malt	safflower,	wheat-free soy
yinnie syrup	cold pressed	horseradish,
		sauce
		lemon
		rice vinegar

Any other food that is not specifically listed in the earlier pages or circled on this list should be avoided until you determine your status at your next consultation. Bring a copy of this list so you can check off your allowed foods.

In general, the healing phase requires reduction in beans, oils, and nuts. You will temporarily avoid oats, salt, fish, spices, buckwheat, noodles, corn, raw salad, fruit, flour products or excessive liquids. Gomashio, umeboshi, miso and seaweeds plus at least twice weekly nishime cooking (using little water, see A. Kushi's **COOKING FOR HEALTH: ALLERGIES**), and ume sho kuzu (ibid.) are helpful. But if you are having too many discharge symptoms, cut back particularly on miso and seaweed. Vary your cooking methods (steam, boil, bake, stir-fry, nishime and later raw); buy as organic as possible, do skin brushing, and see accelerated detox procedure in **WELLNESS AGAINST ALL ODDS.**

Organization is easy if each time you enter the kitchen to prepare a meal, you simultaneously focus on the next 2 days or 6 meals. Organization is simple when you realize it's a tool of perspective or focus. Don't get so narrow that you only see the work of the meal before you. It could have been much easier at dinner time if you had, for example, cooked your rice while showering and having breakfast.

And each meal need not incorporate, as you see, the whole G., G. and B. scenario. That is to help you remember all the items you have available. As I prepare a meal and recite that, it reminds me to add the beans that I have hidden at the back of the refrigerator, or to add seaweeds at the beginning. It's to make life easier, not rigid. Breakfast can very well be left-over rice and bancha tea, only. Or it may be miso soup with or without any grains, greens, seaweeds, or roots.

If you ever find yourself in a panic asking "What can I eat?" Remember: When in doubt eat vegetables.

SUGGESTED MENU

For breakfast:
 The squash drink with veggies and a bowl of grains

(add greens, gomashio, and miso soup if you have time).

For lunch:
Take rice balls or nori rolls and steamed greens, and other veggies including roots.

For dinner:
Grains, greens and beans, roots, sea vegetables and squash as well as condiments. Do not eat within 3 hours before bed, as healing is done at night and you do not want to waste part of that time in digesting. And chew thoroughly, as this promotes assimilation and absorption.

Teas may be taken throughout the day, but in general limit your intake unless you are thirsty. If very thirsty, rinse the salt from the seaweeds (and sauerkraut) or cut back on miso.

Adjuncts:

breathing exercises	positive imagery
yoga, shiatsu	herbal baths & compresses
spiritual reassessment	therapeutic touch
chiropractic	homeopathy
meditation	electro-balancing
gratitude	acupuncture, acupressure

Practice makes everything easier. Consult the cookbooks when you're bored and ready to grow. And remember there is no right or wrong, merely a relentless quest for improvement.

You'll feel the need for condiments eventually. Most are made with miso, soy or tamari sauce and are in Esko's two cookbooks. Besides, gomashio to sprinkle on rice or grains, you can make sea vegetable powders early on when you can't yet tolerate the ferments. They are also rich in minerals. Simply roast kombu or wakame, for example, in the oven at 50 degrees until crisp, but not burned. Grind it in the suribachi and serve. Also they can be mixed with the gomashio.

Onion butter or carrot butter would be good for lunches as a spread. Put 1 tsp sesame oil in a pot, add 10 diced onions (or carrots), saute 5 minutes until translucent. Add a pinch of salt and just enough water to cover, cook on low a few hours until dark and sweet. You may need to add water occasionally.

You can mash any bean or left-over vegetable to make a spread. Chickpea dip or spread can be made in a variety of ways, as can many vegetable dips. Cooked beans can be pureed with finely diced onion, parsley and pitted umeboshi (plums). Or for hummus, add tahini (1:8 ratio tahini to chickpea), garlic, lemon juice, parsley and a pinch of salt.

If your grains or beans become dull, cook them with kombu (acts like MSG as flavor enhancer) or onions. Don't be afraid to experiment once you know your temporary limitations and have read a couple of cookbooks for a basic feel.

Lunch no longer needs to be limited to grains and greens, or nori rolls or stew. You could lightly steam vegetables (keep them crisp) and make a bean dip (water-sautéed onions, mashed with beans, sesame and garlic. This could contain herbs, oil, other veggies, seeds, etc. as desired or allowed.) You can create bean or vegetable pates (use millet "bread" as vehicle; many ideas in **MACRO MELLOW**).

171

If you're too strapped for work lunch ideas, don't push yourself. Slide backwards into a transition diet and use rice bread (yeast free), Essene bread or rice cakes for a while.

SUMMARY

The night before you are going to begin, soak your beans and sea vegetables. Then the next day spend one hour to dry roast your sesame seeds, cook your rice and cook your beans. Now you have these 4 backups. All you do at a meal is steam some root vegetables and greens, and VOILA, you're eating macro. Organization is the key.

DIET SUBSTITUTION STAGES

Note: MB = Macrobiotic

Avoid (standard diet)	Transition (not MB, but getting there)	Healing (restricted temporarily until you are well)	Maintenance (includes all healing foods)
white bread	rice cake	organic brown rice	MB breads, pastas, grains
French fries	organic corn chips	barley, millet, ltd. oats	corn, soy, etc.
cheese	yogurt	seaweeds	tofu
coffee	herb tea	bancha tea	many MB teas
meat	fish, fowl	beans, fish	tempeh

172

sweets, snacks, cookies, cakes, candies, sodas	fruits	squash drinks, pumpkin seeds, boiled and peeled almonds	see MB dessert books, fresh fruit, popcorn
sandwich	yeast free rice bread, sprouts, avocado	nori roll, millet "bread", vegetable spreads	cabbage rolls, MB breads + spreads

Avoid	**Transition**	**Healing**	**Maintenance**
Iceberg lettuce & tomato salad	romaine, all veggies	steamed kale, collards, onion, daikon, carrot, squash, Brussels sprouts, lotus root, parsley, watercress, dandelion, carrot tops, scallions	pressed or raw salads, blanched veggies
ketchup, mustard, mayonnaise, Hollandaise		gomashio, chickpea miso, wheat free tamari, ginger,	herbs, MB pickles, sauces, MB dressings, garlic
cream sauce		kuzu	tofu, kuzu, agar-agar sauces
processed, fresh frozen, canned fried in hydrogenated oils and butter		organic water sautéed	organic limited amount unrefined sesame or olive oil

You see from the above that there are 3 ways to enter a MB healing diet:

1. Jump in.
2. Ease yourself in via a transition.
3. Ease yourself in via MB maintenance diet.

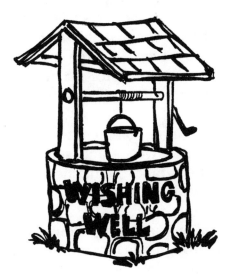

At this point, if you're wishing you had never picked up this book, maybe you're not committed enough to your health at this time.

However, if you're wishing you could hire a macrobiotic cook, then keep going — you'll get there, without one.

GETTING FURTHER ORGANIZED

Tools you will need to purchase right away are a good pressure cooker (Aeternum is a good model with safety features so it's less likely to explode in your face), a strainer, a chef's knife as well as paring knife, sprouting jar and an assortment of at least three stainless steel or glass frying or boiling pans, with covers, a large and small colander, tea strainer, a grater, and a dish for making gomashio: a mortar (and pestle) called a surinami (and surikogi).

Also, you'll want large gallon size glass jars to store the grains, beans, and seaweeds and smaller ones in which to store the teas. Remember grains need very dry storage or mycotoxins can result.

At this point you're wondering about backing out. I know, because I went through this for several weeks, wondering if I was doing the right thing. The foods were so strange, some of them smelled like swamp water. The recipes looked terribly uninviting and some of the compresses that I was instructed to use were so bizarre I was hysterical with laughter. You must be sure to leave time each day to do some yoga stretches or skin brushing to stimulate the circulation. Meditation is also important, but more so is to nurture your spirituality. If God is your co-pilot, change seats!

So let's regroup - you now have bags all over the kitchen of strange looking things that you're not exactly eager to eat. First, you need to organize:

1. Clean out your cupboards. Get glass containers and group beans, then grains, then teas, then sea vegetables.

2. Cut up veggies for squash soup and start cooking (carrots, onion, cabbage or daikon, and squash).

3. Cook up some brown rice. (1 ½ cups spring water to 1 cup brown rice, pinch of salt or 1" piece of kombu. Bring to boil. Put heat dissipater under pot (if you have one) and simmer at lowest heat 45 minutes. Let off steam from pressure cooker and fluff with fork.)

4. Steam some kale or collards (takes 3-8 minutes).

5. Soak kombu and chickpeas to cook later or tomorrow.

6. Give yourself a pat on the back, you have really accomplished a great deal. When you see that there is nothing you cannot do, it will fuel you to continue to learn more. The better and easier your cooking becomes, the more you will do it. The more you eat, the better you may feel and the faster you'll heal.

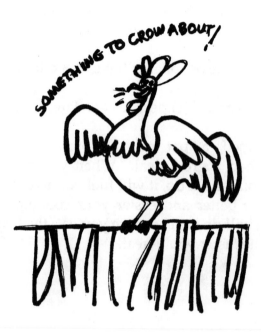

Hey, you're doing great, you can make squash soup, brown rice, greens, beans, and miso soup.

At mealtime, just remember these rules:

1. "Grains, greens, and beans". If you must omit some thing, make it the beans.   50-50, 30-70, or 60-40% are all acceptable ratios of whole grains to vegetables depending upon your condition.   50-50 is safer for starting if you have not yet had a consultation.   And if you tolerate no grains, it's obvious: eat veggies for awhile.   You may require even further modification.

2. If in the beginning the formula seems too difficult, temporarily consider that "Greens" could really mean all vegetables in general, in which case they could be 5-65% (preferably 45-55% of each meal).   Each day try to get these five types of vegetables: **greens** or green vegetables (either kale, collard, mustard, dandelion, parsley, water-cress, scallions, romaine, etc.), **above ground veggies** (squash, cauliflower), **below ground** or root veggies (turnip, burdock, onion, carrot, daikon), **sea veggies** (hiziki, wakame, arame, kombu, nori), and **dangling** veggies or beans (lentils, chickpea, lima, azuki).

3. After a few months, or as soon as you tolerate it, get some ferments each day (miso, tamari) and (macrobiotic) pickles.

4. Watch your overall percentages.   In the first few months beans should be only a couple times a week for allergic people.   Then when they become daily, never should they be more than 15% of a meal, covering less than 1/5th of the plate. Likewise, seaweed should constitute 5-15% of a meal.

5. At each meal be sure to check if you need to have

something soaking (beans, seaweed), cooking (grains or beans), or sprouting (alfalfa) for the next day. A note about chewing: Each mouthful should be chewed at least 50 times. You are eating 50% starch and the digestion of starch begins in the mouth with the admixture with saliva.

So to reiterate, when breakfast rolls around, you could eat your precooked squash soup, add your rice and beans, top it off with a couple of sheets of crumpled, toasted nori (hold over high flame until it turns green) and add diced collard greens and scallions. Cover 5 minutes while steaming. Put some miso in a bowl, add some of the cooking water to dissolve it; add the dissolved miso to the soup and mix. You are ready to serve. I've repeated this intentionally, since this seems to be the most common stumbling block. Macrobiotics is not just a diet, but getting into the diet is the most difficult part for most.

Once you have made the basic G, G, & B in less than an hour, you are on your way to being able to create really interesting and tasty dishes.

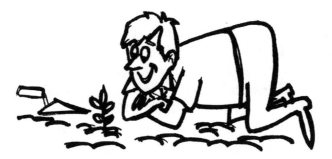

Start an organic garden:
(1) It is good exercise,
(2) it gets you out in the fresh air,
(3) it's satisfying to watch things grow,
(4) it will provide you with inexpensive organic produce,
(5) and it brings you close to nature and our roots.

You could get a hot plate at work and a teapot for mid-morning and afternoon. Occasional boiled almonds, daily nori rolls, occasional mugwort mochi and grated daikon and tamari could be a snack. For lunch you could bring more of breakfast. By dinner time and weekends you'll start exploring the recipe books or have your same basic meal, perhaps just varying it with different seaweed, grains, beans, and veggies. The concepts are balance at each meal. Watch your percentages—on the average, grains 50%, greens 25%, and all else falls in the remaining slot (beans, seeds and seaweeds, roots and "fruits").

You can vary the ingredients or even rotate. You will eventually get into other menus, but I had personally lived this way for three months. I was never hungry. I did have to work at keeping 120 pounds, whereas before I had always been 10 or 15 pounds overweight and could never budge them without a great deal of effort. They slipped off effortlessly the first two weeks and during the whole time I felt well and satiated and didn't get my afternoon slump. I had started healing.

For travel, nori rolls with tiny pieces of umeboshi (plums) and steamed scallions and carrot slivers cannot be beat. You could actually live on this for three or four days. Boiled almonds and steamed vegetables with beans and grains can also be made up ahead of time for travel. Bring some dry roasted pumpkin seeds, too. You could also make steamed leaves rolled about grains for travel (similar to cabbage rolls, only you'll use steamed kale or collards).

For dining out, stuffed squash and nori rolls can be made ahead to take to restaurants. Bring a bancha tea bag so you have something to sip as you enjoy the company...your main reason for being there. You can sometimes order a dish of steamed greens. Or when you're out in restaurants, order a small portion of fish, and a large double portion of steamed vegetables. You can decide if you want raw salad without dressing and their bleached white rice or not. I like to sneak nori rolls into my pocket and let them magically appear on my plate. This balances the rest. As more people request whole foods, more will be available. And remember attitude, a sense of humor, and enthusiasm for wellness are crucial.

Each person would benefit from a counseling session for their specific condition and follow up is crucial since living organisms are not static. You will change, and your needs will change. Regardless of how great you feel at any point, the pendulum will eventually swing. Remember the difference between corrective and maintenance levels for nutritional corrections? A corrective prescription was necessary to correct you. But if kept up beyond the corrections, you created new imbalances. And so a maintenance level was needed. The same applies for macrobiotics.

Remember back to the people with Candida problems? As soon as they eliminated ferments and processed foods and sugars from their diets, many started feeling wonderful and had more energy than they had had for years. But because they were eating such an unbalanced high meat diet, eventually they started going downhill months or years later. This is because the pendulum swung too far in the opposite direction (and many had never corrected undetected nutrient deficiencies or lowered their total load sufficiently). There is a never ending need to assess balance with where you are in regard to diet, environment, nutrient status, symptoms and the rest of the total load.

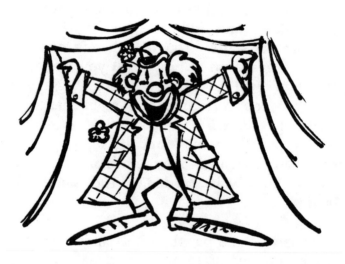

Are we having fun yet?

People eating out of balance will present with the classic problems that tell you they are eating out of balance: (1) they don't feel as good as they did before, (2) they need to be very strict, for if they cheat they feel awful, and (3) they have terrible cravings. Conventional medicine has no concept of this. Cravings are a symptom of imbalance. Dietary needs are not static. Good balance is crucial for constant wellness, and periodic assessment assures we are eating at the fulcrum. Even eating macrobiotically requires assessment due to your changing needs and seasons.

Follow-up Questionnaire

Periodic assessment is crucial for success. Before each follow-up consultation copy and fill out the following questionnaire. In this way you will be able to concentrate on your real needs and not get lost in the details of daily living. Bring this completed form to each follow-up visit. Many will want to copy the first version and merely add to it for subsequent visits with different colored ink.

Name_____

Date_____

How long have you been practicing macrobiotics? _____

What were your primary six symptoms and reasons for doing so?
1._____
2._____

3._____

4._____

5._____

6._____

What have you accomplished thus far?

_____

_____

_____

_____

_____

What remains to be accomplished?

_____

_____

_____

_____

_____

Have you had any discharges? _____
How many?_____

Describe the most pertinent:

_____

_____

_____

_____

_____

Were blood tests done for any of these? _____

What are 4 average breakfasts like?
1._____

2._____
3._____
4._____

Four lunches?

1._____
2._____
3._____
4._____

Four dinners?

1._____
2._____
3._____
4._____

Four snacks?

1._____
2._____
3._____
4._____

What are your general percentages like?

_____
_____
_____

When were your nutrient (vitamin, mineral, etc.) levels last checked?_____

What adjuncts have you evaluated, duration and results?

_____
_____
_____

What MB books have you read?

_____

_____

_____

_____

How much weight have you lost?_____

Check the percent improvement you've experienced during the following intervals since starting macrobiotics:

	Worse	25% better	50%	75%	100%
1st month	____	____	____	____	____
2nd month	____	____	____	____	____
3rd month	____	____	____	____	____
4th month	____	____	____	____	____
5th month	____	____	____	____	____
6th month	____	____	____	____	____
other	____	____	____	____	____
1 year	____	____	____	____	____
2 years	____	____	____	____	____
other	____	____	____	____	____

Overall, what is your assessment of macrobiotics for you?

_____
_____
_____
_____

What are its drawbacks for you?

_____
_____
_____
_____

What would make MB easier for you?

_____
_____
_____
_____

Other comments:

_____
_____
_____
_____
_____
_____
_____
_____

Are you using any injections, supplements or medicine?

_____
_____
_____

Are you using any herbs? _____

Homeopathy? _____ EAV?_____

Besides the diet, what else are you doing for yourself?

_____

_____

_____

_____

How much exercise do you get?

_____

_____

_____

_____

What is the problem for which you have come for today?

_____

_____

_____

_____

_____

_____

_____

_____

_____

Have you consulted a counselor?
Who?_____
When?_____
Advice _____

_____
Result?_____

_____

ARE YOU FEELING OVERWHELMED?

You should be. You're making a major lifestyle change so you can determine if macrobiotics feels right for you. And because of individual biochemistry, no one can give a blanket diet that would fit everyone. But we can give you a general overview that could be modified or adapted to the needs of many. If you don't fit into this scheme, you'll need an individual consultation. Whether or not you need it initially, you should have one within the first three months to check many aspects of your program to optimize your quest for wellness.

As with the Candida and rotation diets, this entails much work on your part. Reading, studying and practice are necessary. More important are the psychological blocks that a person unknowingly thwarts his own efforts with. Because of all of these factors, more than ever we must make it clear that the phone is not the place to bargain for foods or to go over your diet questions. Do not call the office regarding your diet. Re-read this book and schedule a formal consultation (phone or office) where an in-depth evaluation can be made.

If you're having a bad reaction, schedule immediately. If you think you are merely discharging, you may want to get a blood test only. If you have a few well-thought out questions that require short answers, print or type them double spaced on a large paper with enough room after each question for a reply. Include a self-addressed stamped envelope.

A logical beginning is to learn to cook organic brown rice and steamed kale. Substitute if food intolerances exist. You could live on this a few days as you slowly introduce squashes, carrots, onions, and other greens. Next begin to learn to cook beans so that within the first weeks you have grains, greens and beans. You should get your seaweeds, roots and seeds (gomashio is a good first item or roasted pumpkin seeds) in during that time. Miso may not be tolerated until after several months, but periodically (every 2-4 weeks) give it a try.

Your meals can have many formats: the casserole method described combines everything in one bowl. Or you can separate things as individual dishes. As you begin to add other grains and greens, veggies, and seaweeds, you can even rotate if desired. You can vary your cooking style as well: pressure cooking, steaming, stir-fry with water, baking, etc.

Once stuffed squash, nori rolls, casseroles, and individual dishes having been accomplished, you'll be ready to devour the cookbooks for ideas. You'll even come up with handy ideas that are not in the most popular books. For example, millet cooked in the same grain/water proportions as rice (2:1) in a pressure cooker for 40 minutes comes out like a firm bread. It's so firm it can be sliced and used as a vehicle for many spreads like mashed beans or veggies. Later on when you can have oil, it can be sliced and sautéed like tofu. There are many sauces that can be added, like a green sauce of scallions and kuzu. For larger slices, cook millet in a covered saucepan and firmly press it into a loaf pan while it's hot. Slice when cool.

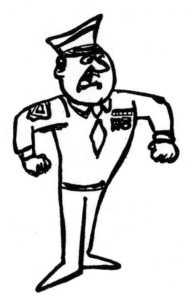

Don't be too tough a task master on yourself. You can only do what you can do. You'll eventually reach your goal if you are determined enough.

ATTITUDE

Obviously, if you thought the four day rotation diet was impossible, or even just the rare food diet, you should not attempt macrobiotics. Also, it should be quite evident that if you do not have cooperation, approval, and loving help from a spouse and relatives, your chances at success are minimal and it will only create tremendous friction. If you moaned and groaned your way through rotation, don't even think of attempting macrobiotics. And don't try to cram macrobiotics down everybody's throat. You're the one who is sick and willing to do it. Loving support is all you can expect from family. Rarely will anyone benefit from a therapy that is forced upon them. When one is sick enough, perspectives have an amazing way of changing.

People often question after they've read something like Sattilaro's book, "Why doesn't the American Cancer Society or the American Medical Association recommend these treatments?" The reasons are very simple. First of all, it's a rare doctor who knows anything about them. Much of our medical education is funded by pharmaceutical companies and macrobiotics does not make any money for them. Second of all, many people will not follow up and consult with the physician, so that he does not keep learning from seeing hundreds of people struggle through these conditions. There is a need for documented studies, but instead people go off and do it, never teaching us about it. If a doctor saw several patients a week who were steadily improving resistant conditions with MB, he'd get very interested. Third, most people would just plain not do it; even some people with cancer would not be able to change their lifestyles to the extent that macrobiotics requires. So, by all means save yourself a great deal of aggravation and possibly even a divorce by not even attempting it, unless you have made a commitment to yourself to take a couple of years out of your life to devote to the pursuit of a new level of wellness.

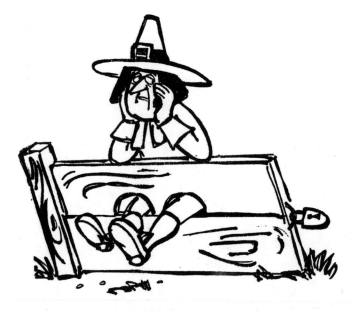

If you feel that your social life is cramped because of macro, you need an attitude and organizational reassessment. Call your macro buddy for help with a creative solution.

If you think you can quietly factor it into your lifestyle without anyone else knowing, think again. You must be prepared for all of your friends and relatives having to make adjustments to your new lifestyle, because it will involve everyone in some way or another. Everyone that is a part of your normal and loving life, that is.

In the first few months you probably will not have any social engagements, or if you do, you will take all of your food with you, as I did. Also, you will not travel or you will, as I did, take all of your food and cook it. A travel picnic cooler is a very handy item to have as well as several wide-mouth thermoses and covered dishes. It can become extremely socially limiting if you don't maintain organization and a good sense of humor. Many of us cook double, in other words we make regular meals for spouses, children, friends and relatives, and our own meals for ourselves. The next 2 books, **MACRO MELLOW** and **THE CURE IS IN THE KITCHEN,** cover more of this.

We realized we had to show people how to dress up their macro, for example, for the teenagers. So we wrote **MACRO MELLOW** which I wanted to call "What to Feed the Rest of the Family Who Hates Macro". And remember that often a mere change of proportions plus the addition of some meat will do the trick. For example, you add hamburger to the meals for your carnivores. And they might have 5-10% of your grains, greens and beans, while your proportions are quite different (and minus the hamburg!)

Not having fruit the first few months is not easy. Furthermore, the smells of some of the seaweeds cooking have been described as "low tide", and that's being courteous. When your whole house smells like this, it makes you have second thoughts. You may spend two to three hours (if you're not organized) cooking and cutting each day. You will need to plan your meals and your time much more carefully than you ever did before, and it's not just a diet change; it's a lifestyle and an attitude change. There is more to improved health through macrobiotics than can be put in one book. It is not merely a diet. But more of this in **THE CURE IS IN THE KITCHEN** and **WELLNESS AGAINST ALL ODDS.**

But in spite of all this, macrobiotics makes so much sense biochemically, and it has such a remarkable track record, that it certainly seems worth a try for many who have nowhere else to go. But I must stress from the outset that, if you're going to be the least bit depressed, or complain one iota about it, you probably will not make it and you shouldn't even attempt it. Fortunately for most of us, we started feeling so good, so clearheaded and so much more level in terms of emotions, and we started having so many symptoms melt away, that we were able to maintain an optimistic attitude and sense of humor. Never once did we have to get angry or militant or defensive. Nor did we have to get on our little soap boxes and start teaching everyone. This is the type of attitude that you must have; if you don't think you can handle it, don't even try. When you're ready you'll know; and when you hurt enough, nothing is impossible.

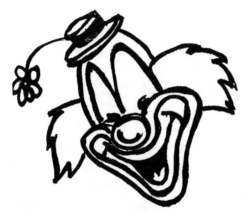

As with all life, a sense of humor is most useful. How can you flood yourself with damaging emotions like anger, frustration, and depression when you're laughing.

While making one of my fuzzy seaweed medicinal teas, that smelled like low tide at Nantucket, I began thinking how important a sense of humor is for enabling one to adapt to this new lifestyle. I thought maybe that was how people were cured of cancer through macrobiotics. They actually laughed so much that they spurred the immune system to new heights of adaptability (ala Norm Cousins).

Meanwhile, in a matter of weeks, strange smells were filling the house. Bags of black and green seaweeds greeted me in the pantry. My nails and knuckles had been grated down to a stage of blood and bones as I was learning to grate daikon and ginger. What remained of my hands was nearly burned off while toasting my nori sheets. I had yellow teeth from my safflower tea, a sunken chest and face from my weight loss and scars on my wrists and fingertips from trying to cut through rocky hard squashes.

I had burned so many grains in learning to use the pressure cooker, that I was on a first name basis with the fire department. Our smoke alarm became the dinner bell. But I can honestly say, through it all I enjoyed every minute and found lots to laugh about. The thing is I felt so much better than I had in years and here I had already thought that I had arrived; that I could feel no better. For indeed through ecologic management, I had attained such undreamed of levels of wellness, that I dared not hope for any more. But macro took us even higher.

Just think how much simpler this whole experiment in health would be if you could choose a macrobiotic selection in any restaurant or airplane. That day may come.

Attitude, especially a sense of humor, and a loving spouse,

are beyond a doubt the primary ingredients to this program. The nuts and bolts you can get from reading and studying and you will have to do a great deal. What we provide here is rationale, motivation, and an organizational guideline to help you get started. You will need to come in for counseling and /or referral to suit your individual needs if you are going to try to maximize your program.

This book was written in an attempt to bridge the gap and ease the transition for you. You will get maximum benefit from it if you highlight and mark pages liberally for your own reference and review. And use blank pages in the back to make your own index.

And remember, there is no medical treatment that has more than tripled the survival from "incurable" cancers that can rival the macrobiotic program (AMER J CLIN NUTR, Carter, et al, 12:5, 203, 1993). It offers hope after medicine has given up hope. And if you fail at macro, there is still hope (WELLNESS AGAINST ALL ODDS). And if you fail there, there is still hope (DEPRESSION CURED AT LAST!). And there are books in progress if you fail there. So never give up; there is a continual avalanche of options.

Try to resist converting everyone. If they're interested, they'll ask you.

HOW TO MAKE MAXIMUM USE OF THIS MANUAL

1. Start on the diet. If you have questions, do not call the office, except to schedule a consultation. We will see you any time you need. If there are questions, reread the manual and also read the other recommended books. You are too individual for short phone communications and relayed messages; they do not accomplish nearly as much as a one-to-one confrontation. They just allow you to slide into dependency and not read. And as they do not allow for in depth dialogue, the answers and conclusions may be erroneous. For every question you ask, we may have six questions that we need the answers to in order to provide you with the best solution. However, if you're fairly certain your questions are straight-forward and require no interaction, write them to us as described and send them in with a self-addressed envelope.

2. For your first consultation, bring a copy of the Diet Questionnaire and have it filled out before your visit. Also bring a copy of Food Choices.

3. Once you have started the diet, always bring a copy of food Choices and the Follow-up Questionnaire. After you have filled it out the first time (having been on the diet at least one month), you can make extra copies of it and merely add to it using different colored ink to update it for subsequent visits.

Having your questionnaires ready saves a great deal of time. Instead of asking you all these questions and waiting for you to formulate your reply, we can get on with the more creative aspects of your individual program, thus you will get to higher levels of accomplishment quicker.

CHAPTER VIII

WHERE'S THE BEEF? QUESTIONS AND ANSWERS

Q. What is macrobiotics?

A. Macrobiotics is a way of life that attempts to harmonize with nature and not fight nature or drastically alter her while adapting to modern technology. Macrobiotics recognizes that a person's health is foremost determined by what he eats, but also by how he eats and cooks, as well as his thoughts and his surroundings. It extends to all levels of a person from his individual person to his family, friends, community, nation, world, God and his relationship with all of these.

Q. My spouse doesn't want anything to do with this. Shall I just go ahead anyway?

A. As with E.I., love and support of your spouse are crucial. I can't tell you how my heart soured when my husband repeatedly insisted that I just do what I had to do. I wrestled with the guilt for a long time and vacillated, cooking him "regular" meals, then, "healthy", and then macro (none of which I do well). He was and is an absolute saint. Don't think it's easy - I was still wrestling with guilt in the fifth month and he lost over 30 pounds! You'll need to experiment with what's best for you. Love conquers all.

Q. How far do I need to go? Do I have to learn all that yin and yang business?

A. That is an excellent question and I do not have an answer. Having read widely on macro and talked with many "converts", I have mixed feelings. As with any endeavor there are those who feel it's an all or nothing phenomenon. But if one studies macrobiotics, you see wife beating, for example, is advocated. I sloughed this point off, thinking it had obviously changed since it was an old print book on macro philosophy. Then I read the 1988 Macromuse issue which featured George Ohsawa's 90 year old widow, and learned she still advocates this! There were other statements, like she would work until he would tell her to rest (not until she decided she needed to rest). This negates the concept of individual biochemistry for starters.

In other books, hairiness in women was considered a bad health sign. Oriental women, regardless of diet are notoriously non-hairy (in family practice I've had the opportunity to examine over 10,000 bodies). At a macro talk two women supported the fact that indeed they had less hair after macro but they were both blonde (a sector of the populous with less body hair). But the French or Italian lass?

Some macro's may feel we're raping their name and using only what we want without understanding the total philosophy (much of which is quite beautiful, actually). In that case, I made a mistake by giving credit to the source of my ideas. I should have pilfered what I could use and taught it under the guise of a modification of the rare food diet (see **THE E.I. SYNDROME, REVISED**). For that is indeed what it is. It's a whole foods, peasant type of eating, devoid of commonly ingested antigens. There is no milk, no wheat, eggs, corn, citrus, coffee, chocolate, beef, sugar or processed foods. And it does pay attention to biochemical balance better than any other diets I have encountered.

But I have chosen not to do that, and instead I have chosen to promote macrobiotics as a modality for healing for people

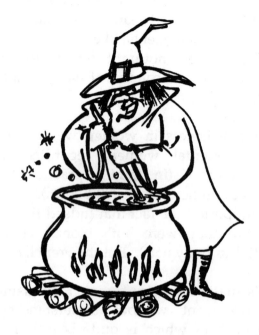

Macrobiotics is not a cult, not a religion, not a form of sorcery. It merely is a way of life that attempts to harmonize with nature.

who have exhausted everything else. Clearly there are, however, stages or levels of involvement in macrobiotics and many may never choose to or need to become total converts in order to benefit.

The yin/yang as the Chinese knew it was reversed by Mr. Oshawa years ago. When foods are cooked a certain way they are said to become more yin or yang. Even long-time macrobiotic people cannot agree on whether a specific food is yin or yang. And since there is no proof and no yin/yang meter, this business discourages many who could have benefited from the rest of macrobiotics.

As you'll see in the next chapter, learning acid and alkaline and yin and yang is important to your success in being able to balance yourself. But no diet is perfect. Critics argue that macro is too high in salt, too low in precious oils (that govern the integrity of all cell membranes, for one), low in B12, too rigid, too unadaptable for western man, etc. But these items can all be monitored and overcome.

Q. I have heard that a macrobiotic diet is deficient in B12. Is this true?
A. No. Just think about it. How could people more than triple their survival with macro and clear end-stage cancers with a diet that is supposedly B12 deficient?

The sea vegetables are a source of B12 and scientific papers bear this out. (AM J CLIN NUTR. 47:89-93, 1988, Specker et al). Also, we have measured the B12 levels frequently in people on macro and if they are following the recommended sea vegetables (specified in THE CURE IS IN THE KITCHEN), we have never seen a deficiency. But you must have either meat, fish, fowl, sea vegetables, or ferments as a source of B12.

Q. How do I select a macrobiotic counselor?
A. We are constantly evaluating them for their effectiveness
   with patients. When I called the Kushi Institute, I learned
   there are four levels of certification. There are no
   counselors within a 200 mile radius of the office who have
   the top three levels of certification. That is why we offer
   our own counseling. That also is why, if you want us to
   be part of your care, you should send us a written copy of
   recommendations from your session with your counselor.

However, remember that many people in the diagnostic
mode, and that includes macrobiotic counselors as well as
doctors, get easily hung up in one area. You know there are
some doctors who do environmental medicine who think
every patient has Candida or every patient has to get rid of
the gas in their homes, and likewise there are macrobiotic
counselors who are familiar only with the old standard
diagnoses of heart disease, cancers, arthritis, etc.

Some are not aware of the problems and intricacies of E.I.
They have probably never seen such profound nutrient
deficiencies as we have documented in patients with E.I., and
they are probably not aware that many of us have
sequestered many chemicals which may take years to
depurate or detoxify; and this may retard healing immensely.
Healing can likewise be retarded indefinitely in a too
chemically contaminated environment for that individual.

It is easy to appreciate how a counselor can become over-
confident after seeing an end-stage cancer victim heal. It is
understandable why the seemingly less life-threating
complaints of someone with E.I. would give him/her a false

sense of security. This is precisely why many with Candida, leaky gut, intestinal dysbiosis, and chemical and food sensitivities have been made seriously ill. For this reason we counsel our patients or will recommend the best counselor that we can. It's a tailor made decision.

As a test, I saw two different "counselors" and their diagnoses were 180 degrees out of phase. And I've been in a room full of counselors where they could not agree. There is no substitute, therefore, for knowing as much as you can. Two excellent books for starters would be **ACID AND ALKALINE** (Herman Aihara) and **FOOD AND HEALING** (Anne Marie Colbin).

Q Why is meat so bad?

A. In olden days, a festival or feast was a rare occasion for a celebration. All the stops were pulled as the banquet tables were prepared. Now we are such an affluent society that we feast every day. Not only is a diet high in amino acids too acidic (requiring too much buffering), but on a worldwide view it makes even less sense. It takes 30 times more grain to raise one beef, compared with the number of people that can be fed with that same grain. And animals concentrate pesticides many fold. But the immediate problem for meat is with its high acidity. For example, someone with serious liver or kidney disease must restrict protein, whereas grains are sustaining. This is because in a weakened condition some of the buffering mechanisms are already malfunctioning. Why stress our bodies unnecessarily on a day to day basis and over-work our marginally operating buffer systems? Save it for a feast or special occasion. Baskin-Robbins Ice Cream heir, John Robbins', **A DIET FOR A NEW AMERICA** will give you more reasons to avoid meat than you ever

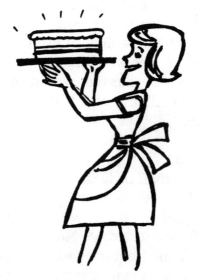

If you're still having cravings, you're eating out of balance.
Don't suffer; let's find out what's wrong.

dreamed of (1-800-847-4014).

Q. How do I know if I'm getting enough calcium if I'm not drinking milk?

A. You can get just as much, if not more, calcium from an equivalent amount of greens such as collards, kale, and watercress, also almonds, and many other foods. Colbin's **FOOD AND HEALING,** and Aihara's **BASIC MACROBIOTICS** are some of the many books that will give equivalents of many of the nutrients and nutrient values of many of the foods. Remember when we lectured in China for a month in 1985, we never had or saw any milk or cheese, and they do not have nearly the osteoporosis incidence that we do in this country. For one, the Chinese tote home bundles of fresh greens under their arms each night. But in the U.S., we're not big greens eaters. Two, most of our foods are processed which means they have high levels of phosphates which inhibit the absorption of calcium. So we have two major mistakes. Next, high acid (meat, soda and sugar) diets pull calcium out of bones in order to buffer the acid. Also calcium absorption depends on proper stomach acid, which many are deficient in, and significant portions of accessory minerals (boron, magnesium, etc.) have been removed from processed foods, but are necessary in order to put the calcium in bone. When these minerals are missing, we instead put calcium in artery walls, which is why arteriosclerosis is the number one disease.

Q. Should I go off vitamins when I do macrobiotics?

A. This is individual and you should discuss it with the doctor. Basically, macrobiotics does not recommend vitamin supplements. However, many of the people that we see are extremely low in certain nutrients. We have

211

watched macrobiotics correct nutrients, but it has taken, oftentimes, six to twelve months to do so, and it might be better to correct yourself in a month or two and then discontinue so that you have a "head start".

Don't forget that macrobiotics is a very old healing philosophy, and it is learning to modify and adapt to newly created 20th century diseases, such as E.I. and the multiple deficiencies that we have caused through our way of processing foods and our changes in dietary habits. The chemical environment has definitely created new and unheard of problems with newly formulated chemicals of every description in people's bodies disturbing the normal biochemical function. Macrobiotics is in the process of adapting. For example, many of us are exquisitely sensitive to natural gas, and of course, macrobiotics recommends the use of natural gas over electrical cooking because of interference with electro-magnetic fields and vital life force energy in foods. Many of us must cook with electric (and have healed with it). For many I would never recommend returning to gas.

Furthermore, this century with unprecedented exposures to daily chemicals, forces us to detoxify them. In the process of detoxifying our daily exposures, we use up many nutrients. There is tremendous loss of nutrients in the work of detoxication. I suspect this is a major reason why some long-time macrobiotic people have even developed cancer.

Q. Should I go off my injections when I'm on macrobiotics?
A. Again, macrobiotics would say go off them as soon as you can. However, we have a specifically weak population that is genetically susceptible to developing chemical hypersensitivity. Furthermore, hidden nutritional

deficiencies can promote the spreading phenomenon leading to further sensitivities to foods, molds, Candida, and other chemicals.

Many needed titrated allergy injections a while in order to keep the total load sufficiently low enough to be able to cope. Some need them indefinitely. Remember, not everyone may do their program as perfectly as they need to for their condition and macrobiotics isn't some magic cure-all. People have developed cancer while they were on it and died. So your best bet is to stay on injections at the interval you need to control symptoms until you see the doctor. The idea is to get your total load low enough to allow your body to heal itself. Many will go on monthly injections and hold it there for a couple of years. Then if you decide to abandon macro, or your symptoms worsen, all you need do is go back to once or twice a week. It will save you re-testing.

For some, their total load is just plain too high and they need injections to help reduce it. It is one part of the total load over which they have control; and there are too many other areas over which they have no control.

Q. What if my chemical sensitivities get worse on macrobiotics?

A. That would be quite possible, and we have seen this in environmental medicine with a mere diet change. Sometimes it's a loss of adaptive enzymes or an unmasking that causes this. The problem is in deciding whether it's an actual discharge reaction or a real worsening of chemical sensitivity. You should see the doctor when this happens. It will help us learn about your individual system and whether your liver is really discharging. We may even be able to measure some old

213

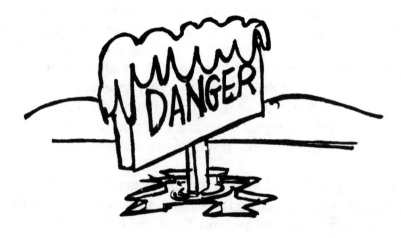

When in doubt, see the doctor.

chemicals (pesticides, drugs, formaldehyde, etc.) as they come out of the fat storage into the blood on their way to the liver. For others, you may have finally reached bottom in some nutrients that is crucial to detox. We can measure this. Or you could start by having your family doctor get the blood levels recommended in **TIRED OR TOXIC?**

A discharge usually fulfills the following criteria:

1. It is preceded by your feeling great.
2. There is sudden development of symptoms, but there was lack of the usual trigger.
3. The symptoms many times are bizarre and things that we have never seen before.
4. During discharge symptoms, there is often a strange feeling of "It's O.K.". The victim does not feel compelled to rush to drugs as in the past. Instead, he feels content to let the body do its thing and clean out.
5. The symptoms should be gone within days or weeks. Past a month, I would not consider a discharge as the cause and would recommend a through medical evaluation.
6. Once the discharge is over, you are left feeling that you are now at a higher level of wellness than before.

Q. How can I tell if I'm having a discharge reaction or symptoms?
A. The best way is to see the doctor and/or have some blood work done. Bear in mind that when one is having a discharge, there is often a certain mental set where even though you're having symptoms, you may have mental clarity which normally you would not have during these symptoms. You also have an unprecedented feeling of well-being or peace that you normally would not have with these types of symptoms.

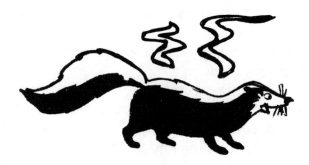

When you are discharging you will, from time to time emit horrid odors. You might as well prepare your friends. I thought maybe they didn't notice. I was wrong.

Q. What if I need to take medication?

A. Macrobiotics attempts to detoxify the system and get rid of chemicals, just as we also try to keep people free of medication in environmental medicine. If you must take medication, however, do so; especially if you are a severe asthmatic. Never hesitate to take your medication if you feel you need it. Varying amounts of time are needed for people to heal sufficiently without their medications. Never risk making yourself dangerously sick. And when in doubt, see the doctor.

Q. What if I need to stop my macrobiotic program?

A. Once you have started you should decide on a commitment for a specified period of time, usually six months. If you stop and start, you may make yourself worse, and at best you will slow the healing process so much that you'll become disenchanted with the whole program and discontinue it. When in doubt, if you get caught in a bad situation, in a restaurant, order only steamed vegetables or mineral water or just don't eat. Bear in mind, carbonated waters are not desirable, as they deplete body buffers in the process of neutralizing the carbonation (carbonic acid).

Q. What if I lose too much weight with macrobiotics?

A. Weight loss is to be expected, and you will lose in the first few months, and should. People will be telling you that you look awful and you should eat more. But just remind them that you're getting rid of old fat and chemicals, and then you're going to put back your fat again, but with clean, organic foods and you will only be putting back as much fat as you actually need. If you find you have too much weight loss and cannot control it, you should see the doctor. Another clue that the weight loss is not detrimental is if you are feeling great.

Q. What evidence is there for macrobiotics?

A. There are many scientific papers on macrobiotics. Some references are in Michio Kushi's **THE BOOK OF MACROBIOTICS** (1987). Also see our book, **TIRED OR TOXIC?** which gives over 30 biochemical mechanisms in lay terms (and with references for physicians) that explain why it is so healing. And for even more evidence, see **WELLNESS AGAINST ALL ODDS** and the books and the newsletter that follow (this same publisher).

Q. Will I need my Nystatin and Vital Dophilus to treat Candida on macrobiotics?

A. Remember, Candida is merely a symptom that you're not biochemically balanced. It signifies there is still a stressor present and you are not playing with a full deck. Once you have a healthier body, you'll be able to go off the Candida program and not have the symptoms. For example, you can take an antibiotic and not get Candida once you are healthy. Many people do. Also remember, that a vast majority of the people with Candida are better right away, just off sugar. They have quickly relaxed their buffering system and removed one of the major drains on the system. Remember, too, meat keeps the sweet cravings alive.

Q. Should I rotate on macrobiotics?

A. Yes, you should, but in the beginning you'll be lucky to just do macrobiotics, much less rotate it. However, after about the sixth month, you'll probably be infinitely more sophisticated and able to rotate. I suspect we all should do that and macrobiotics does stress a varied diet. Remember, we still are part of the 21st century where we are capable of becoming sensitized to foods that we eat repeatedly. Ours is a genetically weaker and chemically more stressed breed of people than has ever been studied before.

A horse, for example, is a huge and powerful animal. Yes it lives on 95% timothy hay and alfalfa with 5% oats, corn, and a salt block. Man has distorted his diet and environment to foster the development of the leaky gut (see **WELLNESS AGAINST ALL ODDS** and subsequent books). This is a major cause of food and chemical allergy which necessitates rotation.

Q. What if macrobiotics isn't working?
A. You should see the doctor and make sure you're doing things correctly. Some people do better with a tailor made program that is not in the 50:25:10 percent ratio for G, G and B.

Q. What if I don't tolerate any grains?
A. This often happens with people with severe E.I. You may need to start with non-grain carbohydrates such as quinoa, amaranth, tapioca or buckwheat. Also, you may want to fast for three or four days and then try oats, barley, organic brown rice, or millet and see if you tolerate those once you are unloaded. If not, you'll need to go to the greens, squashes, and beans for starters. You'll most likely benefit from counseling help. Some need food injections and leaky gut tests. Also see ideas in **THE CURE IS IN THE KITCHEN.**

One universal reactor was bedridden with pain and exhaustion when she was referred by the medical center.

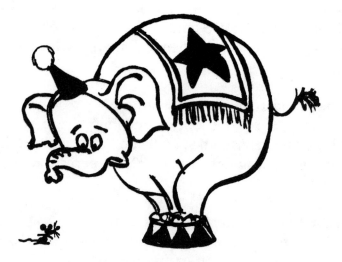

Weight loss is effortless with macrobiotics. If you are normal or underweight to begin with, you will need closer supervision.

On the E.I. program she made remarkable improvement in her previously severe chemical sensitivity and Candida problems. She was out of bed, caring for the family and household. But just the smell of fabric softener sheets from neighbor's clothes dryers as she walked with her children could trigger symptoms. She decided to go the next step and eat macrobiotically. But she developed severe exhaustion as though there were a severe deficiency. However, she found the solution in eating broken grains. In other words, by grinding the grains into flours and making pancakes, she began deriving relief from more E.I. symptoms and without the weakness. Clearly she has a digestive problem, possibly resistant Candida, like the dreaded C. tropicalis (see **THE E.I. SYNDROME, REVISED** for explanation) from using Nystatin too long.

Q. How important is it to phase out my injections under medical supervision?

A. Very. It may be the difference between struggling through a tough discharge of weeks or months, or sailing through a mild one. Most of us who work cannot afford to take off several weeks to be ill.

First, remember that some people we have seen could not even begin to clear in the first place on macrobiotics without reducing their total load (see **THE E.I. SYNDROME, REVISED** for explanation). This total load included chemically less-contaminated food and air. It also includes pushing the body to make blocking antibodies and T suppresser cells to turn off an abnormal reactivity to air borne molds.

Secondly, there is the question of immunologic memory. When someone gets measles or the immunization, they usually have lifelong immunity to it. The body remembers to produce those antibodies for years to come. The immunologic memory is good. With tetanus, flu and other immune stimulators there is varying individual response. Some people remember to make antibodies for years; others only a few months. If you have poor immunologic memory for allergy injections, within 2 years of stopping, your symptoms will recur.

Remember, a carefully titrated allergy injection contains nothing more than what you would normally breath anyway: It's just in a route and dose that stimulates your body to produce the helpful or blocking antibody (IgG) as opposed to the harmful one (IgE). In general, each person is highly individual and should assess this with the doctor to minimize having to retest at some time. Some people will require a periodic reminder to boost the immune system, others will not. As long as it's there to keep the body unloaded enough to get on with the work of healing, that is all that matters.

Q. What about some of the herb baths that are recommended?

A. Again we must balance 20th century "faux pas" against benefit. Most municipal U.S. waters contain levels of chlorine that make many people with E.I. ill. To deliberately immerse your body in it if you know you react is silly. There are a couple hundred other chemicals in it as well. Chloroform and trichloroethylene can be volatilized just from the shower spray. You will need to assess your severity of sensitivity and the degree of contamination of your water to decide if the benefits of the baths outweigh the risk.

Q. What if I don't tolerate any foods?

A. You may need to start on food injections and a rare food rotated diet in order to be able to tolerate foods. Then you can gradually swing into a more macrobiotic routine. Go back and assess your total load and follow the E.I. checklist. If you're too chemically overloaded, you'll never tolerate foods.

Q. What if I get worse while I'm on macrobiotics? What if I get very ill, have excessive weight loss, feel awful and have constant symptoms?
A. Then you should see the nurse counselor or the doctor so that it can be determined why you are worse. You should also check that you are chewing your foods well, that you have the correct proportions, and that you are not overeating. Also, be sure that your foods are mostly organic, and if you are still having trouble, you should definitely see the doctor.

Q. What if I am having chronic diarrhea?
A. When in doubt see the doctor, especially if it persists beyond 2 weeks. You can get dangerously depleted of potassium and/or magnesium and precipitate cardiac arrhythmia which could be fatal.

Q. What if I feel macrobiotics is against my religion?
A. There are theologians of nearly every persuasion that are among the macrobiotic community. Macrobiotics is not against religion, and it should not interfere with yours.

Q. How long should I stay on macrobiotics?
A. At least until you are well, then I would be very cautious about modifying. I would suggest you read **Wellness Against All Odds** or Colbins', **Food and Healing,** and try to modify in terms of these, rather than returning to your

canned fare. Hopefully you will have learned so much about yourself that you will not really abandon, but merely modify.

Remember some people get dramatically worse once they veer from this program. This is partly because of loss of adaptation. A first cigarette makes one ill, the second is better, and the rest is ancient history. Actually it is wonderful that you feel sick in a newly painted room. Who wants a blood stream with carcinogenic volatile organic hydrocarbons in it? Just because others may have adaptive enzymes that allow them to tolerate such exposures doesn't make them any less resistant to the potential long term effects like E.I., hypertension, arthritis, hyper cholesterolemia or cancer, as examples.

Q. What if I hate the food?
A. If you don't feel peaceful and serene on the program, I would suggest that you visit a macrobiotic center and have some of their meals. You might also have meals prepared by others who cook well macrobiotically, and determine if it's your neophyte cooking that is uninspiring. There are several good macro cooks who will cater; try them out. Also, be sure to check your proportions or balance. And then again, remember that macrobiotics is not for everyone, nothing is. **WELLNESS AGAINST ALL ODDS** spells out the alternatives.

Q. What do I do when I want to go somewhere?
A. You must plan since the average American cuisine is not healthfully oriented. I usually had some umeboshi-nori rolls or boiled peeled almonds or roasted pumpkin seeds ready so that I could dash off for several hours, and if I ended up in a restaurant I would have something to

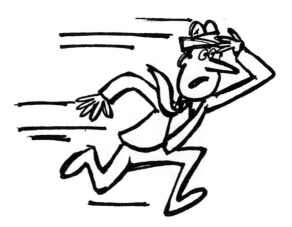

Diarrhea is a common discharge symptom. When in doubt, see the doctor, especially if it lasts more than 2 weeks.

nibble on.

Q. Why don't I just go vegetarian?

A. There are many vegetarians who are extremely unhealthy. Many of them are overtly obese. Some of them are very vitamin depleted. This is because many of them are not knowledgeable about good nutrition and under the guise of not eating meat, they eat a tremendous amount of wheat products often flavored with honey. They also tank up on broken grains (breads and pastas) and have far too few sea vegetables which supply minerals and B12. However, on an airplane or in some restaurants, vegetarian would provide a partial substitute for you and be far better than all the dairy, meats, and processed foods that you would get in the normal restaurant fare.

Q. What if I modify the macrobiotics?

A. In the first three to six months I would not modify anything, because you are trying to see how much of your symptoms you can simmer down with a program that has taken years to work out.

Q. Why are there no famous octogenarian macrobiotic people?

A. This question bothered me, as well, for I know many leaders in the field of clinical ecology who are in their 80's and appear healthier than many people in the 60's. But I have not seen this in macrobiotics and it disturbs me. I hope we will have an answer soon. Lima Ohsawa (wife of Georges) is 90 and in admirable condition. He, however, died before 70. In John Robbins' book, he lists famous macrobiotic athletes.

Q. What do I do if I feel my program doesn't have much

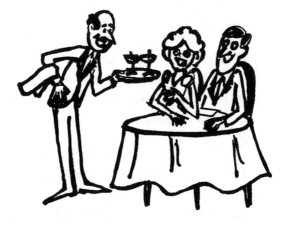

As long as you pay attention to your stage of treatment, you can go anywhere. You just need to realize what you can and can't have. Then it's simple. You know right away if you should bring your own food or not. Remember you're going for the social fun, not the actual food.

supervision?

A. Schedule by phone or in person to see the doctor or the nurse counselor so that the program details and your questions can be dealt with fully.

Q. How do I make my journey to wellness go faster?

A. Many things will slow you up. Probably the best things to speed you up will be to eat less and lose more weight and generally eat 50-60% rice. Moderate exercise, more sea vegetables and miso, sweating, massage, ginger compresses, meditation and other adjuncts also aid to speed things up. And, of course, keep your life ecologically clean. If you are overburdened by a chemically contaminated environment you may forever retard healing.

Q. How do I know if I'm doing things correctly? Does anyone make house calls?

A. At this point we don't have anyone that does. Your best bet would be to write out your menu and proportions of foods that are ingested for each meal and then share that with your counselor or the doctor.

Q. Could I die from macrobiotics?

A. I have never heard of this happening on the diet outlined in here, but if at anytime you just plain don't feel well, you should see the doctor. An examination plus specific mineral, vitamin, amino acid, essential fatty acid, and other blood tests can be checked. Perhaps you have a deficiency that's been unrecognized in the past. If anything should kill you, it's what you have eaten in the past! And, there is always a possibility of developing a new condition for which modern acute care medicine is

After you're well, then you can add fruits and desserts. For healing purposes they are too yin or expansive. If you have doubts that you're getting sufficient vitamin C, let's check it out with a blood test. My motto: When in doubt, check it out.

suited.

Years ago some people died who stupidly ate only brown rice. That scenario has become a legend among people who malign macrobiotics without fully understanding it.

Q. Could I get deficient on macrobiotics?
A. Yes, but only if you do it incorrectly. Macro stresses variety, just as we in environmental medicine stress rotation. It gives you much more variety and less chance of developing deficiencies than does the S.A.D. (Standard American Diet). When in doubt, we should check your levels. Good indicators of your status would be a vitamin A, B-carotene, 1-OH vitamin D3, B12, C, and RBC zinc, and RBC: magnesium, copper, chromium, calcium, molybdenum, potassium, manganese, and selenium for starters.

Q. When do I branch out?
A. After you have gone through a couple of discharges and you have vastly improved some of your major symptoms, then you can start eating a more lenient diet. Your goal is to get well first.

Q. When do I have my first steak?
A. Possibly in a year, possibly never. It depends very much on the person and his needs.

Hopefully, with your macrobiotic reading and experimentation with the diet, you will see that you feel better than you have ever in your life, and it will change you so that you will never be the same again. The same thing happens with people who go through the rare food, rotation diet to identify food allergies and learn about processed foods

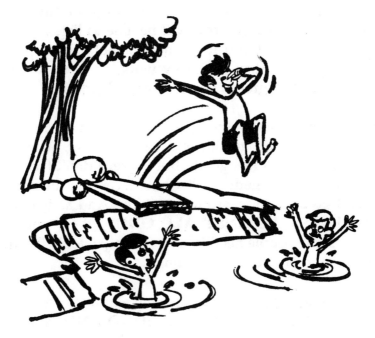

Exercise is important:
(1) it helps detoxify,
(2) it helps stave off depression,
(3)it improves body tone, and
(4) it adds to your confidence and
concentration.

and nutrient deficiencies. Even though they may not stay on a rare food, rotated diet all of their lives, or they may not stay on a Candida diet all of their lives, they have learned so much that they could never go back to the junk food life that they had had in the past. They are forever changed or altered for the good. When you are healed, you will have steaks and assess how you feel. You will be able to listen to your body and determine if you need meat or not. Some people must have it. Either they do heavy work, or work in the cold, or get so bland on greens that they bore themselves.

I used the macrobiotic diet and got rid of literally every symptom. I can go out and have a steak, wine, chocolate mousse, etc. and feel great. But if ever I don't feel 100% well, happy, and energetic, or if I have even the tiniest symptom, then I go back to macro for a while. And as you will see in **WELLNESS AGAINST ALL ODDS**, there comes a time when some people need to go off macro for a while. Our bodies and environments change.

Q. What do I do if I am fantasizing about ice cream?
A. Anne Marie Colbin's book, **FOOD AND HEALING**, has many suggestions for cravings; umeboshi (plums), "rice cream", amazake and better balancing of your diet are some of the many things that can be done when you have cravings. Remember a craving is a good thing; it is a clue that you are out of balance. It is a warning before illness and degenerative problems occur. Severe sugar cravings can signify something as simple as a chromium or manganese deficiency.

Q. Do I need a buddy?
A. Absolutely. This makes everything in life easier. If you can find someone who is going to go on the program with

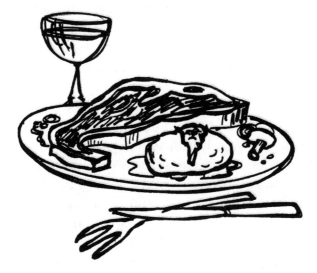

Some people need meat. Some people don't. It's very simple, if you just listen to your body. But you'll grossly distort its signaling system by feeding it plastic food.

you, that you can confer with each day, that you can share expenses when you buy bulk at a co-op, that you split up shopping chores with for strange items, it always makes things easier. Also, it's always nice to have someone that you can laugh with.

Q. How long should I let bad symptoms go on?
A. No more than two weeks if it's a bad symptom such as chronic coughing or congestion, or achiness, or mild diarrhea. If something like asthma or diarrhea is very bad, you may only be able to let it go a day or two, then you should be checked to determine if it's a discharge phenomenon or not.

Q. Why don't I just stay on the same diet that made me well?
A. Because the pendulum will always swing to the opposite side sooner or later and then you'll feel lousy because of what you're eating. In other words, take people who have Candida. They feel wonderful in the first few weeks or months when they get off so many sweets. Then the pendulum swings to the opposite end where they are having a proportionately larger amount of meats and they begin to feel lousy because of this. There is no diet that is great for everyone, and likewise even when a person finds a diet that is great for him, it does not mean that it will remain great for him. Through all levels of stress and environmental conditions, his needs change, his seasons change, his body changes. The diet that makes you well, is not necessarily the one that you should stay on. Besides, the diet that makes you well is usually quite restricted, and the diet you want for maintenance is infinitely more varied and lenient.

Remember, when we correct vitamin deficiencies, we first put

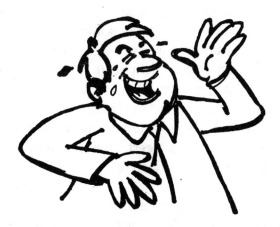

A buddy is indispensable. It's much more fun to have someone to laugh with. And as you both devour the more advanced macro books, you'll teach one another.

people on a corrective supplement program which is extremely unbalanced, but it must be unbalanced to balance the extreme imbalances of the deficiencies. If we leave people on this corrective program, however, they will develop other deficiencies once the first ones have been corrected.

Q. What do I do about going out to dinner?

A. There are many things you can do. You can call ahead and make sure they have some brown rice and some steamed vegetables for you. You can bring some of your own little snacks. You can order them at a local vegetarian cafe and take them with you. Don't forget, restaurants are in the business of selling food. They adapted to the needs of clients with high cholesterol and diabetes. If there's a need, they'll adapt to the call from those eating macrobiotically.

Q. What do I do about airplane travel?

A. There are three possibilities. One, you can fast. Two, bring your own food. Three, you can order vegetarian and pick through and maybe be able to find a few nibbles that you can tolerate. Your best thing is just to bring your umeboshi-nori rolls, since the umeboshi can help balance the inhaled xenobiotics.

Q. What do I do about vacations?

A. Since I am the universal guinea pig, I went on three trips out of the country in the first four months of my program and took all of my own food. I also took some to restaurants; it can be done. I have one suitcase with a hot plate, pot, spoon, grater, sea vegetables, etc.

Q. What happens if I eat meat or fruit or sweets, bread, or ice cream?

A. There are a number of things that can happen. One, you can slow up your program. Two, you can create an imbalance that will then trigger other cravings. Three, you can set your progress back for weeks. Four, it means you missed a marvelous opportunity to learn how to correct an imbalance that you had, since uncontrollable cravings mean there is an imbalance that needs correcting.

Q. Should I keep a diary?
A. Yes.

Q. Should I put my family on the diet?
A. It all depends on how eager they are to do it. I would not force it on anybody. Oftentimes, you can ease the foods into the meal plan and frequently people will become interested when they see your wellness materialize. **MACRO MELLOW** helps make your food look more like "regular" food.

Q. How do I know I've detoxed?
A. You'll know because you'll feel better and better after each discharge reaction and have progressively fewer symptoms to endure as you tolerate a broader range of exposures. But don't push yourself too fast. Just because you are less reactive, don't over-expose or test yourself and deplete your detox nutrients. Allow the body to continue to heal and see just how well it can get.

Q. What if I get severely depressed or irritable?
A. This may be a symptom or a discharge and you should see the doctor when you're in doubt since blood tests can be done to discern which is present.

Q. What do I do if I get severe pain or severe weakness or

severe weight loss?

A. See the doctor when in doubt.

Q. Why are the men in macrobiotics so skinny? No wonder they're all pacifists. I need a diet to suit my build.

A. There are robust macro men, but yes many are slight of build, and I don't have an answer. I suspect the answer lies somewhere in the fact that oriental men are often of slighter build than some other nationalities. Therefore, modification of the diet may be in order for some nationalities.

It's ironic that Ohsawa lectured in France on macrobiotics telling them to eat by the laws of nature and the foods that were indigenous to the area. No wonder many ignored him. How much daikon, wakame, rice, and miso are indigenous to France? There are apparent incongruities. All I know is there is a system here that works well for healing, and that it can and must eventually be modified for use by greater numbers.

Q. Are macrobiotic foods irradiated?

A. That's a tough question. Proponents of food irradiation try to get away with as little labeling as possible and increasingly more items are being OK'd for irradiation. As you know, the process destroys a significant portion of vitamins and creates new untested chemicals called "unique radiolytic products" (U.R.P.). They are not something conducive to healing.

Q. Is mercury toxicity a problem with the seaweeds?

A. I don't know, but it's one of the minerals we'll be investigating as we assess people eating macrobiotically. A 24 hour urine for mercury before and after 4 weeks of

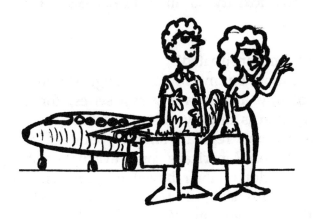

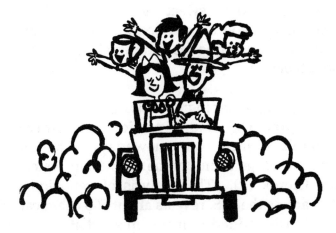

Vacations, large or small, just take more planning. There are publications you can order that give locations of vegetarian/macrobiotic restaurants and services all over the world. You could always bring brown rice and have your hotel cook it for you (or bring a hot plate and cook your own when you need balance).

sea vegetables should tell you. The protocol for testing for heavy metal toxicity is in **WELLNESS AGAINST ALL ODDS.**

Q. What if I'm constipated?

A. Constipation on macrobiotics suggests the need for a colonoscopy and bowel X-ray series, for correction of constipation is usually one of the first benefits. Movements become regular, simple, painless, and odorless; whereas most Americans could evacuate a shopping mall with the odor of their bowel movements. Constipation suggests putrefaction in the gut. Toxins will be absorbed into the blood stream. If your bowel movements are not daily, soft and sweet smelling (unless you are discharging), you should see the doctor. You may have something a simple as intestinal dysbiosis, which is correctable.

Q. Can I use tap water in my cooking?

A. No. Most U.S. municipalities have way too many chemicals in their water nowadays. The chlorine level some mornings at my home in the tap water smells like pure Clorox (R). The analysis of xenobiotics for many cities across the U.S. reveals about 500 chemicals. Some are intentionally added to mask others that are too expensive or impossible to get rid of. Industrial contamination of water tables is rampant in the U.S. Many of the chemicals are hydrocarbons which, of course, are free radical sources. In other words, they create naked electrons that dart around aimlessly leaving destruction in their

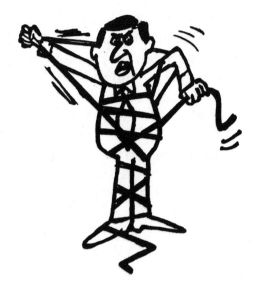

If you're not happy on macrobiotics, you'd better see your counselor or the doctor. You may be eating wrong.

pathways. The membrane and protein destruction that results can potentate aging, allergies, degenerative diseases, mutation and cancer (see the **E.I. SYNDROME, REVISED**).

Q. I hesitate to ask but, how do you cook brown rice?

A. Most of us did not know. There are many fine cook books and courses, but to speed up your initiation: Wash 2 cups of brown rice in a colander, sort for stones, put in pressure cooker. Add 3 cups clean water, a pinch of salt, and turn on high. In about 5-10 minutes the whistle will blow. Put heat dissipater between cooker and burner and turn to the lowest setting for 40 minutes. When timer goes off, remove from burner, prop fork under vent to let off steam. Fluff with a fork. Voila!

Q. What if I just have too many food allergies or macro bothers my stomach?

A. You need a test of whether you have the leaky gut syndrome. It can cause food allergies and make many foods intolerable. If it is leaky, then you need tests (CDSA and purged parasites, Great Smokies Lab, 1-800-522-4762) to determine if unwanted organisms are causing the leaky gut. Details of the diagnosis and treatment are in **DEPRESSION CURED AT LAST!** (this publisher and author).

Q. I've eaten according to Macro rules and I don't see any difference.

A. No one therapy in the world is for everyone. But the most common reasons for failure are not watching the proportions, (see **THE CURE IS IN THE KITCHEN**), having poor environmental controls (see **THE E.I. SYNDROME, REVISED** and **TIRED OR TOXIC?**), and failure to reduce stress. The latter should include an enjoyable exercise program, meditation, reflective lifestyle modifications, a spiritual reassessment and self-nurturing. You must start doing loving things for yourself and others each day. Or you may have a much tougher problem and need a combination of techniques described in **WELLNESS AGAINST ALL ODDS** and **DEPRESSION CURED AT LAST!**

Do a periodic attitudinal assessment. See food as a friend, as a positive healing tool, not as an enemy and something that will bring on reactions. Find out what's really bugging you in life and get rid of it. Many people harbor subconscious insecurities, anger (which fosters guilt) and hurt which keeps "eating at" them. These demons must be devoured so you're once more as mentally free as a child. Only then can your playful, creative, and loving instincts emerge.

Rx: Bring laughter into your and someone else's life every day.

Q. Now that you are into health, does this mean you trade your high heels and suits in for construction boots and long skirts?

A. There's much to be said for a back to nature lifestyle, stress reduction, non-conformity, and lessened obsession with obtaining all the accouterments of suburban society. But on the flip side, we owe the movers and shakers more than we could ever hope to repay. I hope health will become so "in", that a 3-piece suit does not look out of place in stores where sacks of grains and beans predominate. It is beginning to happen.

Q. How about a quick synopsis?

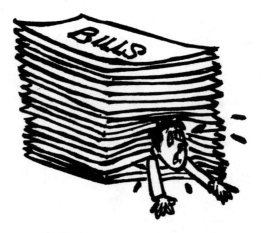

As you will see, you can eat far more inexpensively with macro as compared with the Standard American fare or rare food organic rotation.

A. Cut out meats and sweets. Substitute grains and greens. Work into grains, greens and beans, seeds and (sea)weeds, roots and "fruits". Don't forget miso soup once or twice a day once you begin to tolerate it. Chew each mouthful well. Watch your proportions: 50-25-10% of G, G, and B, or 50:50 of grains: vegetables. Check your nutritional levels. Periodically evaluate your progress with the doctor, and learn what's new on the horizon, as well. Periodically re-assess your goals, short-comings, accomplishments, methods and motivation. When in doubt, check it out; see the doctor if not doing well. Read, read, read and then talk with successful macro people.

Q. I have practiced macrobiotics for years and think you have oversimplified the diet and underestimated the remainder of the philosophy.
A. You're right. Bear in mind we're trying to do the impossible here: (1) Identify a discipline compatible with the discipline of environmental medicine that also can take people beyond what we have been able to accomplish in the past. (2) Having accomplished this, we now need to devise a way to make this foreign and difficult philosophy palatable. In attaining these goals, much has to temporarily suffer or be shorted. If macro is as beneficial as I think it is, it's taking off much too slowly. It has many drawbacks for the yet unconvinced Westerner.

I'm merely trying to show the logic and simplify getting started. If the person starts to get the results he's been looking for, he'll be hooked and go for perfection, learning all he can. Anyone who gets that far has to realize he carries the ball and we cannot spoon-feed him the rest of the way, although we did spell out Mr. Kushi's strict phase healing diet in detail in **THE CURE IS IN THE KITCHEN**. We can

245

match each person with the most suitable counselor, we can help him monitor and modify, but he does the work and must also be constantly learning. Macrobiotics broadens a person's awareness and urges him to explore other alternative therapies if macro does not suit him. As you will learn in **WELLNESS AGAINST ALL ODDS**, even people who are meant to be carnivores do well with 3-6 months of clearing out on macro.

Q. I found the diet to be the least helpful and the philosophy to be my mainstay.
A. True. For some, there is even progressive emotional discharge as they relive aspects of the past.

Q. Isn't it true that one has to embrace totally the philosophy of macrobiotics to get well?
A. There is wide biochemical variability. Some people need meat. There is a wide range of sickness. Many get better with diet alone. That's probably due to the fact that it's the perfect rare food diet and for the most part avoids the extremes of acid/alkaline, and avoids processed foods, concentrating on whole, vital foods. Clearly, the philosophical attitude of macrobiotics provides even further benefit: There is never a reason for anger, jealousy, depression, or self-pity when you believe (1) nothing is totally yang (there is some good in every thing), (2) sickness is a good thing; it's the body's way of balancing or discharging, and (3) you are responsible for your illnesses, but on the other you have the power to heal them. As well, there are many additional benefits that extend to the cosmic man. And, of course, on the other end of the spectrum are many other pluses; seeing food as friend, not as an enemy, living closer to nature so that awareness and appreciation blossom, etc.

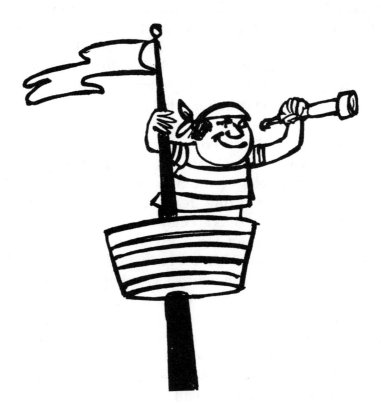

Keep a look out for bum excuses. If you don't have time for macro, maybe you just plain don't choose to make time for wellness at this point in life under any conditions. You're just not sick enough.

Q. I've heard macrobiotics is very strict.

A. I've heard Mr. Kushi teaching a class to aspiring counselors in healing. On one hand, he insists that MB is not rigid, but the broadest, most flexible diet there is, that there are no forbidden foods. And indeed, a wide variety is recommended. On the other hand, he tells them if they eat chicken or meat, or eat "chaotically", such as while working at one's desk, this reflects a shallow life and indicates they are not suitable to be counselors.

Many aspects of the philosophy are right in line with the positive and creative visualization techniques that the field of psychoneuroimmunology would suggest. Symptoms are viewed without paralyzing fear: a cancer is seen as a localization of harmful cells so they can be gotten rid of. All sickness benefits men, for the mechanism of symptoms is to make the patient better. He must have faith in this constant struggle for harmony with nature. We should be grateful for symptoms, or we would have become extinct long ago if we hadn't had a way of discharging our excesses. It is because of sickness that mankind survives. When sickness is seen as bad, he continues, there is no gratitude, no self-reflection to see how you can make yourself better. Macrobiotics fosters tolerance, a spirituality if you will.

But this is carried even further where they are anti-immunization (fine if the whole world is macrobiotic, but if one person is not, he'll start an epidemic, theoretically), no medical system, no military weapons (they feel aggression comes from eating meat), etc. There are many arguments that corporate America could counter with. I'm not certain if one needs to be a pacifist in order to fulfill the macrobiotic ideal. You can decide how much of the philosophy suits you. The peace of mind and faith seem to suit many.

Q. This is ridiculous, how could one possibly hope to heal, for example, a coronary artery plugged by arterio-sclerosis?

A. The medical profession has trained us as physicians to perform more like auto mechanics. We see a malfunction and replace the part. It's easier often than restoring the old. The problem is, your body is not a car.

Our mechanical view is pervasive—if one has a case of bad colitis, cut out the bowel and throw it away (it's practically heresy to look for a hidden food allergy). You have fluids in the ear canals? Anesthetize the little kid, puncture his tympanic membrane and put in a drain tube. Don't look for the most common cause, dairy allergy.

With coronary artery disease the same mechanical view is held when drugs fail. Cut out the arteries and put in some from the leg (bypass) or just ream out the old ones (angioplasty).

A recent publication (**Hospital Practice,** May 15, 1988) by a Mayo Clinic researcher shows there are receptors in those blood vessels that cause relaxation of the vessel when the lining is healed. These very same receptors cause contraction when the vessel wall is inflamed. But what simmers down inflammation more definitively than a search for ecologic triggers and a good healing diet? Furthermore, studies show that flax oil or eicosopentaenoic acid decreases reactivity and inflammation of vessels (see **THE E.I. SYNDROME, REVISED**) more than with aspirin. But this information takes time to reach those cardiologists who are not yet even advocating avoiding all processed foods that contain hydrogenated vegetable oil. They still recommend margarines and egg substitutes containing dangerous trans fatty acids (see **DEPRESSION CURED AT LAST!**) Some of this oil contains coconut oil which is 88% saturated fat (beef is only 40%, egg 33%). It's ironic that the "low cholesterol" plastic foods, like artificial coffee creamers, are actually recommended by hospital dietitians for patients with dangerously compromised coronary arteries. And need I tell you why? Suffice it to say Dean Ornish, MD (Lancet, 1990), has shown that when bypass surgery and drugs fail to control advancing heart disease, the macrobiotic diet has reversed the arterial plugs in one year, proven on PET scans (see **WELLNESS AGAINST ALL ODDS** for references).

Q. How can something you eat affect your moods?
A. There are many levels on which this occurs. First is by a direct allergy, second is by affecting balance and pH, and third by having disharmonious electromagnetic frequencies. Also, there are receptors for many intestinal messengers, like vasoactive intestinal peptides in the gut, lung and brain for example. All the data is not in, but clearly reactions in the gut are transmitted to brain receptors. Lastly, there is the psychogenic taste and gratification aspect. There are over a dozen mechanisms for food-induced reactions (see **DEPRESSION CURED AT LAST!**).

Q. Can zinc deficiency cause AIDS?
A. It is interesting that most AIDS victims in whom an RBC zinc is tested are deficient. Zinc is crucial for synthesis of a thymic factor whose deficiency does contribute to the syndrome, AIDS. It certainly could be one of the vulnerability factors that set the stage.

Q. As a physician who studied over 9 years, and practiced over 26 years, how can you recommend something where lay counselors diagnose such idiotic things as mineral deficiencies without so much as a blood test?

A. Much of it I agree, does sound bizarre by our standards, but when you observe people, for example, having elevated liver enzymes when they are supposedly going through a liver discharge, it's mighty convincing. Much is common sense, however. For example, they look at fingernails for splitting and breaking, hair for dryness, frizziness and breaking and suspect mineral deficiencies. They add more seaweeds and the nails and hair change in 6 months. Doctors could do this as well, especially since they have all the tests of proof available to them.

I have witnessed a skilled counselor diagnose liver problems in a nurse with normal liver chemistries. The diagnosis was made by noting the faintest yellowness in the medial sclera (whites of the eyes on the nose side). And the counselor was correct since the nurse had just gotten over a severe case of shingles that had caused severe pain in that area.

What gets me is how was all this was figured out years ago. They go further and attribute specific emotions to specific organs: anger for the liver, fear for the kidney. And darn if it doesn't pan out much of the time. When patients are no longer as chemically reactive or up urinating all night, those emotions mellow out. I have felt it in myself and observed it in others as well.

In **TIRED OR TOXIC?** we presented 33 biochemical mechanisms for everyone to understand which explains how macrobiotics can be so healing. For example, if one eats meat, there is more of the enzyme B-glucuronidase in the gut. Often the body gets rid of toxic chemicals by carrying them through the bowel and hooking them on to a large carrier molecule (conjugate). It costs the body enzymes to accomplish this, as well as detox nutrients. The problem is that gut B-glucuronidase rips the conjugate off the toxic chemical so that it can be re-absorbed back into the blood stream. So you wasted all that energy, nutrients and chemistry to detox a nasty chemical, only to get it back again. But when one does not eat meat, the B-glucuronidase level is very low, so bad chemicals are not re-absorbed and the efficiency of detox is improved.

Likewise, macro has maintained for years that fruits are too yin and expansive and weaken the liver through their watery nature. Imagine my surprise when I found an article in the journal **Laboratory Investigations** showing that intravenous fructose (fruit sugar) in rats caused severe cellular swelling in the liver and damaged the chemical detoxication mechanisms in the endoplasmic reticulum where detox begins. Now how did MB figure this out years before this work with electron microscopes was done? These are powerful observations, the likes of which seem to be a lost art today. (See **TIRED OR TOXIC?** for explanations and references of further examples).

Fascinating as it is, I can't agree with all of it yet. I see myself as a negotiator, merely attempting to get West to look at East. There's no question the West's strength is in acute care medicine and masking symptoms, and the East's is chronic disease and health. Why can't we enjoy the best of each?

Q. My counselor insists I use miso, but it makes my Candida symptoms worse.
A. It should and you need to have a more up to date counselor selected for you. Mr. Kushi in his book, **ALLERGIES**, shows the best understanding of environmental illness I have ever seen by a non-ecologist.

252

So perhaps your counselor has not studied long enough, and for sure, hasn't had too much experience with E.I. or Candida.

When you're well, you'll have no problem listening to your body. You may feel exhausted for example, at a change of season, and find you get a boost from some fish or chicken. You can eventually learn how to eat to feel great all the time.

Don't forget you're in a constant state of flux, as are the seasons and your environment. This requires monitoring and modification. But once you are cleared out, you can rely on your instincts to give you feed back on what is appropriate for you. You'll notice animals in the woods are not sucking down pills, nor walking with canes. In fact, they are rarely sick because they have instincts that we have suppressed. When they are thirsty they drink. Compare this with us, drinking because we are hooked on alcohol, caffeine, or sweets. In fact, we don't even know what hunger is, for we rarely give our stomachs a chance to dry out. We eat foods we are addicted to, high in fats, sweets and salt. And when we have a God-given craving, instead of gnawing on the back of some tree, we forage in the refrigerator for Haagen Daz.

So once you get off these and clear out on whole foods, you'll lose many symptoms that covered up your ability to detect reactions from foods. After all, how could you tell that sugar makes you tired when you were exhausted most of the time before, anyway?

For example, I was full of anger one week, and it just didn't make sense until I examined my cooking and realized I was using too much salty miso and getting my liver too tight. By increasing the greens and backing off the miso, it was easily corrected.

Q. I've heard of people getting cancer while on macrobiotics.

A. Dirk Benedict, a handsome T.V. actor developed his cancer while on macro and cured his cancer by refining his program of macrobiotics (**THE KAMIKAZI COWBOY** is his story). This type of question I do not have an answer for. Then there's a book about a man who had cancer of the pancreas. He cleared on macrobiotics, but he later died of pneumonia. On autopsy they were delighted to report that he died of pneumonia. Why couldn't a simple pneumonia be conquered if progress was so good with macrobiotics that the pancreatic cancer was cleared? Granted everyone has to die sometime.

Q. How much should I eat?

A. You should only eat to about 80 percent of your satiety, especially if you are overweight. The less you eat the quicker you will have a discharge because you will be getting rid of fats which contain many of the xenobiotics (foreign chemicals).

Q. How do you determine if I'm having a spontaneous depuration (detoxification or an actual discharge reaction) or symptoms?

A. Vitamin and mineral levels, enzyme levels of organs, including liver enzymes and a gamma glutamyl transaminase are some of the useful parameters that help us differentiate, and we're working on building a data base that will help doctors differentiate even more precisely in the future.

Q. What if I fail on macrobiotics?

A. There's no such thing as failure and you should avoid

feeding yourself negative vibrations like that. If macrobiotics does not work out for you, it may be that you are a person who does not need it or chooses not to do the program. However, with all that you have learned   and read, I'll bet that you have more whole grains, greens, and beans in your diet than ever before. In other words, once you have passed this way you are forever changed for the better. I for one, rarely had any greens, roots, beans, or whole grains.   Even though I do not remain macro all my life, you can bet I'll have a healthy proportion of them forever.   Most of us had a monotonous diet of bread, cheese, and wine, beef and sweets.   Secondly, none of us did macro 100% well the first time, or the second, or the third. It is a learning and growth process.

Q. What if there's no difference or no improvement after three months?
A. Then you should make sure that you have reduced your environmental load, watched your proportions and checked with the doctor. Read **THE CURE IS IN THE KITCHEN** for details that may enable you to figure it out alone. You may have, for example, serious nutrient or hormone deficiencies, or intestinal dysbiosis (see **WELLNESS AGAINST ALL ODDS**).

Q. How do I know if I would benefit from macrobiotics?
A. You never really know until you try it, but most people are going through life at half mast because they don't really know what wellness feels like. It's much like a child who is born with defective vision. He never knows that the rest of the world sees a much greater array than he does until someone fits him with a pair of glasses. If you don't have a great appetite for simple food, if you can't fall asleep within five minutes, if you don't have a

good memory and a good sense of humor, precision of thought and action, creativity, enthusiasm and freedom from fatigue, then you may find that through the macrobiotic system of eating that you could feel a great deal better. Also, if you need any more than six hours of sleep a night, it's worthwhile to evaluate the program.

Don't forget that conventional medicine only recognizes end-stage symptoms. It totally ignores and even derides the notion that early symptoms or subtle symptoms are of any importance. However, every symptom is a potential warning of more severe problems to follow. Ask any heart attack victim. Most of them just had a vague feeling of unwellness and excessive tiredness the week before they had their grand slam heart attack. And, of course, for years prior to this, they ate the wrong foods and many did not enjoy a fully exuberant state of wellness. If you can't awaken cheery, playful, and laughing in the morning and truly say, "I feel wonderful," then it behooves you to evaluate the macrobiotic way.

Q. How did I get E.I.?
A. There are multiple factors at play in the development of E.I. One is heredity. Superimposed on that usually is poor nutrition from years of eating processed foods or a lot of sweets. Then the detoxification system starts to peter out because of missing nutrients, such as zinc. Then the psychic stage may also be set with all of the mental garbage that we carry around.

Feelings of insecurity, guilt, jealousy, anger, are all very detrimental to the psychoneuroimmune system. Or there can be a tremendous emotional upset such as a divorce or a death, and, of course, there can be the monotonous diet of the same processed foods all the time, eventually triggering the

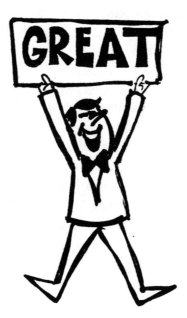

Regardless of whether you become a full-fledged macrobiotic convert or not, by learning about it and trying it you have introduced yourself to a new level of wellness. I'll bet you include more whole grains, greens, and beans than you did prior. Even if it's only once or twice a week, it's better than none, which is what most of us had before. So you can't lose.

upset of the apple cart. Candida sensitivity through many fermented and sweetened foods following antibiotics is a well known trigger. And, of course, many chemical hypersensitivities can start the landslide that we are all so familiar with; a new office, a new home, renovations, and the like. So can the leaky gut trigger it (see **WELLNESS AGAINST ALL ODDS**).

Q. How long did it take me to get E.I.?

A. Probably, much like most other disease, it is something that built up over the years, not something that came suddenly. The problem is that our sudden awareness of the disease only came about because of an eventual collapse of one of our body's systems. For example, it may take 10-20 years to develop a cancer, but you only notice it when bleeding starts or the lump is big enough to feel one day. But the process had been building for years, just as it does in people with heart attacks, arteriosclerosis, diabetes, arthritis, colitis, cancer, etc.

We often speak of a heart attack as some disease that happened in five minutes. Quite the contrary, it had been building a long time. Likewise, reversing the pathology should not consist solely of a quick fix with a pocketful of pills. Healing takes consistent intentional care over a long period of time.

Q. How long do I need to be strict?

A. Until you are healed. You and your physician or macrobiotic guide will determine this. But do not stay strict for over 1-6 months without guidance, especially if you are worse or not changing. When one is healthy, one can eat nearly anything once in while. If you have cancer, I cannot recommend strongly enough at least a week seminar at the Kushi Institute in Becket, Massachusetts. And then I would never recommend that you go off, for every person I know who did, died of a recurrence after they had initially cleared their cancer.

Q. How careful do I need to be about cutting my vegetables?
A. The size and shape effects the cooking time and thoroughness. Even the tools you use are important. After 2 years I purchased a standard macrobiotic vegetable knife (N.E.E.D.S. Syracuse, NY, available by phone 1-800-634-1380 and mail) that changed my cooking. It made much finer slicing available which shortened cooking time and improved the nutrient status as well as taste.

Q. I've read some of the recommended cookbooks, but I need help.
A. **MACRO MELLOW** by our nurse and macrobiotic guide, Shirley Gallinger and myself, may fill the bill since it takes an approach that no other macro book does, spelling out planning, planting, growing, harvest and storage tips. Also included are menus, recipes, and hints for making an organic macrobiotic transition diet for the family.

In fact, you can learn to use your macro ingredients to cook meals for them without their realizing they are eating macro. This helps you better organize in the kitchen, while being able to use the same ingredients for everyone's meals. So this book is for transition and for the rest of the family that hates macro. When you are ready, **THE CURE IS IN THE KITCHEN** is the strict healing phase for you (all available this publisher). **THE QUICK AND NATURAL MACRO-BIOTIC COOKBOOK** by Aveline Kushi and Wendy Esko, (Contemporary Books, NY 1989) is also good for the busy budding macrobiotic.

Q. What is shoyu sauce?

A. The only type of bottled sauce you should use in the healing phase. In the beginning macro was afraid American soy sauce with corn syrup would be used, so they used the name tamari. But when tamari was made in the U.S., it was a by-product of miso manufacturing often with added alcohol like mirin. It is not appropriate for healing and should not be used. Use shoyu sauce (and know your reputable macrobiotic manufacturers and read labels carefully).

Q. Can I add miso and eat it right away?

A. No, it is too tightening and it is best to simmer it over a low heat for a few minutes (2-3). The same goes for shoyu. Do not over cook or cook too high as you will kill the beneficial gastrointestinal organisms.

Q. Can I make soup for every meal and just put everything in it?

A. No. You won't chew your grains well enough. They should be dry for 2 meals, but can be in porridge for morning. Just add water to left over grain and cook 20 minutes, add seaweed or sesame powder (see **MACRO MELLOW**).

Q. There is so much stress in macro books on using a gas stove; should I consider it?

A. I personally would not. Gas gave me terrific headaches, unwarranted depression and back muscle spasm in my 25 year old break. There are those who think some will never heal if cooking with an electric stove. And I would recommend gas to a cancer patient, but not to one with E.I.

or chemical sensitivity. However, many have. You could try a backyard gas barbecue grill for a cooking trial, or buy a small gas unit for the kitchen before making a major switch. See if it is tolerated and improves you over a month or two trial. Many of us tolerated gas after we were cleared, but in this day and age I'm not sure we need an intentional extra load.

Q. How do you know discharges actually occur and that they are not just ordinary illnesses?

A. To give you an example, one gal's hands, liver area and neck area oozed purple that even stained her clothes and bedding. It occurred after nine months of macro, during which time she got progressively better. After two weeks of this she returned to normal, healthier than ever. Purple was the color of the permanent wave solution that she had used with her bare hands on patrons as a hairdresser for eighteen years.

Q. I'm still unclear why cooking methods are so important.

A. Cooking changes many properties of a food. The more you cook, the more digestible, but also the more nutrients that are lost. For root vegetables, large pieces are cut when they are cooked 20 minutes (nishime style) and grated ginger juice added. But fine slices may be used for shorter cooking.

For greens, avoid cooking them past their peak of color. In other words, as greens become greener that is the optimum eating time. Stop cooking here and sometimes you'll even need to rinse them in cool water to arrest the internal heat from cooking them further. Past this point they begin to lose color as well as nutrients.

261

Q. Why did I have to read all that nutritional detoxification biochemistry? It seems like there are two separate books here: one on nutrition and one on macrobiotics.

A. We are the first (experimental) generation of people fed such devitalized foods and simultaneously exposed to so many chemicals. We break all the rules of medicine, and macrobiotics as well. (2) As we realize that the responsibility for true health and healing lies with the individual, we have a further responsibility to educate. (3) Because of these factors, plus tremendous individual biochemical variation and constant new research findings, it appears prudent for each person to understand the need for guidance in monitoring and modifying his program. In addition, the more you can understand about your chemistry, the better chance you have of getting well and staying well. The complexity becomes self-evident.

Q. Since I have E.I. am I more prone to cancer?

A. Usually people with E.I. are more prone to immune diseases such as arthritis, colitis, lupus, multiple sclerosis, and arteriosclerosis, while generally people with cancer and AIDS tend to be on the other end of the spectrum of immune dysfunction. Usually with cancer and AIDS, the T helper cells are deficient. The bottom line is there is no statistical evidence yet.

Q. Why is there such controversy in medicine regarding macrobiotics?

A. As with any therapy that takes control away from the doctor, and that most doctors are untrained in, and that does not make any money for drug companies, it does not receive any medical attention. Therefore, there's no research money. Therefore, there's minimal scientific investigation. Therefore, it is easily ignored and discred-

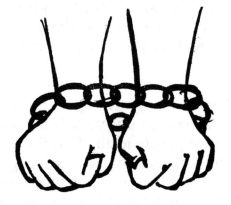

If your hands are tied and you become stuck at a stage with no progress, see the doctor. Keep good records of what you did that brought you to new levels of wellness. They will provide clues to your biochemistry.

ited by those unfamiliar with the scientific proof behind it.

Also, most acute care therapies are proven with double blind tests. This is easy if you're looking at the effect of one medicine. That means neither the doctor nor the patient knows if he is receiving the real medicine or nothing (a placebo or "sugar" pill). Only at the end of the study is the code broken. Hence, double blind studies have become the gold standard. But that's a shortsighted view. How can you double blind the lifestyle and diet changes of E.I. and macrobiotics?

Q. Why are there so many alternatives to health?
A. You're right, there are many roads to "roam" (pardon the pun). I've seen people totally heal E.I. with macrobiotics, with prayer, with divorce, with nothing, with correcting their nutrient deficiencies, with injections to just foods, molds, or chemicals, correction of their Candida problem, colon cleansing, homeopathy, amalgam removal, and all of the above. I know of people who are trying to heal with the Gerson therapy, and I know of people who are much better having had polarity therapy, phenolics, and bio-energetic therapies. We merely began by trying to find something that has a pretty good track record that also is more or less workable for the person with severe E.I. and that makes sense as a stepping stone in minimizing your future health problems. We were looking for something that also could correct the 20th century nutritional deficiencies that constitute an unrecognized epidemic. We also wanted a modality that could detoxify people as well as a modality that was respectful of biochemical individuality and cognizant of the increasing chemical pollutant load. Macrobiotics was the only thing that answered all of these needs. And most importantly, it is a

God-given natural therapy, affordable for anyone.

Furthermore, many of the above alternatives produced only partial and sometimes transient or fleeting results. Macro appears to bring about a much more fundamental and lasting level of wellness.

Q. Why hasn't my doctor heard of macrobiotics?

A. He's peddling as fast as he can. Give the guy a break. In this era there are over 2000 scientific journals to be read. Our input of information has become staggeringly impossible to be of practical use. Why not give him a copy of **WELLNESS AGAINST ALL ODDS** and make it easy on him. Why should he have to spend years "rediscovering the wheel"?

Q. How can I have rice for breakfast?

A. Just as easily as you can have coffee decaffeinated with trichloroethylene, loaded with pesticides, a devitalized sugary donut made from bleached wheat with many additives, or toast made from the same thing, or orange juice from dyed oranges, heavily pesticided throughout their growth cycle. When you think about it, the English breakfast of baked beans or even kippers is far healthier. Basically, you want whole foods that are not devitalized and that have a life force or energy still residing in them.

Q. I've heard you can get really sick if you go off macrobiotics.

A. After 5 1/2 months of macro, I found myself thousands of miles from home in a remote area. After a few days I decided to abandon the hope of continuing macrobiotics while on this trip. At first I tried to eat cautiously, but after a week, my old eating habits were in full swing.

The first thing I noticed was that these old favorites didn't taste as good anymore, and I really yearned for some pure G, G and B (grains, greens, and beans). I also felt like these foods weren't digesting. One day I decided to try a dish of ice cream and succumbed to a three hour deep sleep. A few days later the same treat only caused a 2 hour nap. I was beginning to adapt (masking).

By the end of a week, I had a night of such diarrhea that I didn't have two contiguous hours of sleep. That did it! The hotel would not locate any brown rice for us and they would not even cook it if we brought it to them. There was no alternative. My husband and I set out to purchase a single electric burner. The fifth store we consulted had one for $20.00. Then we sought out the town's only health food store and got brown rice, kale, onions, carrots, Mt. Valley glass bottled spring water, miso and umeboshi (plums). I felt like we had discovered gold. Back at the hotel, I had a sudden blinding headache, and discovered they had started painting the elevator next to our room while we were shopping. We unpacked my other purchases: a covered saucepan, knife, spoon, dish and set to work. In less than 24 hours I was feeling great again. The experience taught me several useful lessons:

1. I was nowhere near ready to expand my diet.
2. Macrobiotics is indeed a powerful healing tool for my body.
3. I would not dream of venturing away from home without all the supplies to prepare my own food until I was very well again.
4. When pressed, we can all accomplish amazing feats.

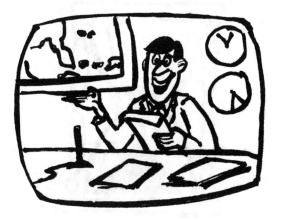

As you've learned through E.I., medical controversy is usually based on money and ego, not science.

If lack of time is your excuse for quitting, why not read Alan Lakein's classic time management book, **HOW TO GET CONTROL OF YOUR TIME AND LIFE.**

I must admit, I'm not the problem solver, my husband is. Had I been alone, I probably would have suffered the symptoms. He, on the other hand, is not restricted by convention and the impossible. He sees every obstacle as a welcomed challenge to his ingenuity and a tool for further growth. It's only too logical to him that if G, G and B are what I need to feel better, then that's precisely what I should have.

Don't lose sight of the fact that negativity and "it's impossible", and "I can't" may be part of your symptoms too. Actually, as I've lectured over the globe, I have met many Orientals who cooked in their hotel rooms. And when the restaurateurs realize there is a profit to be made by just having some healthful, whole unbroken grains on the menu, we will no longer need to carry our cooking supplies.

I realize how absurd our world has gotten when I'm ecstatic just thinking of finding a hotel whose guest room windows open and that serves glass bottled spring water and organic brown rice.

Q. Why do some people have worse reactions than they used to once they veer from macrobiotics?

A. They are unmasked. If your body doesn't like something it gives you a symptom. Many people ignore it or drug it. Or they have so many other symptoms that they don't notice it. Once you're on clean whole foods and start eating junk again, you should feel wretched, as I did. If you persist, however, you can adapt again (but you'll develop other problems). When we give a baby processed food, he spits it back in our faces. We think it's cute and ignore the poor kid and force it down until he adapts.

269

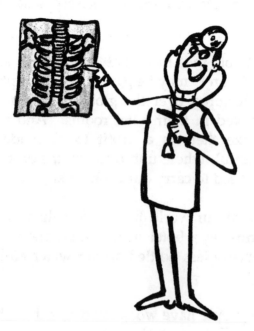

We need good scientific documentation of the effects of macrobiotics. We need to show that you really do detoxify, and correct your nutrient levels. And as we collate this data, we will be able to present it in a way that the scientific medical community can appreciate. It is already happening.

Q. Is it all right if I eat.......?

A. Remember there are 3 diets. A transition (to ease you into macro), healing (individually prescribed and temporarily restricted) and maintenance (full of variety and fun). The maintenance is most liberal to use (once you're clear of symptoms, unmasked and unmedicated). The healing diet is the most restricted and its phases are tailor made to your disease, your general condition, and your monitored response. To plea bargain for foods is to retard your progress. Why not be as strict as necessary and get on with healing, for later you can eat as you want.

Q. I went macro years ago and the counselors made me worse.

A. That's because some counselors may be less experienced or rigid or have not yet adapted to the needs of E.I. The gestalt psychiatrist thinks gestalt psychotherapy is going to help every patient. The same goes for the Freudian analyst, the rational emotive therapist...etc. People get stuck in their own niches where they get the best results. You can't treat a cancer patient the same as an E.I. patient, and further there is tremendous individual variation among people with the same diagnosis. In general, many allergic people do not tolerate grains (especially wheat), nor soy, nor ferments.

Q. When I'm out of town why don't I just go to a Japanese restaurant?

A. Japanese, Tai, Vietnamese, and Chinese restaurants are just about as far removed from macro as the standard American restaurant. Most all of them use devitalized, bleached white rice, hydrogenated oils, and much MSG (which tastes peculiar when you're unmasked). Some are loaded with incredibly hot spices. But sometimes you'll get lucky and find some suitable substitutes. My husband ordered sushi for me on a flight, thinking it resembled my nori rolls; I couldn't resist breaking out in to song, "If you knew sushi, like I know sushi........"

Q. What is hardness?
A. Hardness is a term applied to many of your organs that macrobiotic people will use. When they diagnose you as having a hard liver, for example, what they mean is through years of much yin ingestion, such as sugars or alcohol or chemical inhalation, the yin response of the liver is to expand, become swollen, boggy, and lose its elasticity. Couple with that years of ingestion of fats and salts such as much beef and hard cheeses, and this swollen, boggy, expanded liver becomes filled with mucus and fats which block or impede the energy flow. It can also become a breeding ground for chronic infection. Eventually, it can even calcify, especially if you ingest synthetic vitamin D1 enriched products such as milk. It becomes firmer (hence, hardness) until it is very ill and no longer properly functions. Then it starts adversely affecting other areas of the body.

Q. What is discharge?
A. Discharge is a phenomenon whereby as weight is lost, the pH becomes more balanced and mucus, old chemicals and toxins are presumably pulled out of hard organs and discharged. There comes a time when many of the stored chemicals and toxins are mobilized and float freely in the bloodstream, thereby mimicking the very symptoms that you normally complained of. With in a few days or weeks, when this phenomenon is complete, your health will be at new levels. During this time it is sometimes necessary to fast in order to allow your body to use all of

One of my goals is to remove the isolation that people with E.I. and on macro feel. Making our successes known in the medical literature should bring us closer to a day when you can go into any restaurant and have a choice of macro (just as you now can have special foods for diabetes or high cholesterol).

its energy for completing the discharge phenomenon and not waste any of it on digestion.

Q. What are some of the reasons for discontinuing macrobiotics?

A. People who have discontinued give the following excuses: They didn't have time to plan, shop, and prepare for the meals. Their spouse hated the stuff. They didn't like the smells in the house. They found it very boring. It didn't taste good. It limited their social lives. However, bear in mind that if the norm in a restaurant was that you could find macrobiotic food, it certainly would change things immensely in many of those categories. Also, many of those categories reflect that the person has not had adequate training in cooking lessons, which is essential. Or perhaps they are not yet committed to wellness?

Q. What can I drink?

A. Thirst, like any symptom, is a God-given mechanism for survival. When an animal needs water, it has thirst and searches for water. Man cannot rely on this, because (1) he eats highly salty and fatty foods so he has abnormal thirst and overworks his kidneys by drinking to excess. (2) Man drinks for taste and mood, not for thirst. He drinks because he likes the sweetness and the high from alcohol or a Coke. He has distorted his thirst feedback mechanism.

If one is eating whole grains, greens and beans, they contain over 50% water and very little else is needed, especially when salt is as reduced as it should be. So drink an occasional cup of tea if you need it. Bancha, safflower, or roasted barley are fine. Be sure to use glass bottled spring or well water for all your cooking and teas, however.

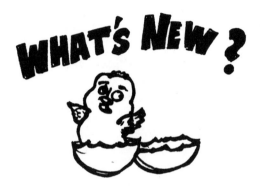

Please check back with this office at least yearly, even if it's just by phone. There is constant newness. By knowing what your current status of gains and problems is, we can help you in your quest for wellness. Also, the newsletter (**TOTAL HEALTH IN TODAY'S WORLD**) will help keep you abreast of new findings.

Q. What if I can't give up coffee, cigarettes, or beer?

A. You are not getting enough bitter greens. These are bitter cravings and designate the need for greens and to cut back on salt and increase the sweets and/or sour.

WRITE YOUR QUESTIONS AND COMMENTS DOWN NOW WHILE YOU'RE THINKING OF THEM........

CHAPTER IX

WHAT NOW?

As you can see I've tried to accomplish a number of items.

1. Top priority is to get people who are still suffering from chronic disease, especially E.I. and Candida, better. (By now you realize that nearly all chronic disease and Candida is E.I.)
2. Help others who are not getting as much out of life as they could to find a new level of wellness, and to prevent future disease.
3. Be fair and open minded about a non-medical discipline yet at the same time maintain some semblance of scientific credibility.
4. Give credit to macrobiotics for this massive contribution.

However, I cannot at this stage support all that macrobiotics stands for.

1. People have developed and died from cancer while on macrobiotics. Like anything else there are no guarantees, except death and taxes.
2. There are many strange sounding remedies like taping an ume plum to your navel for sea sickness, baking some of your hair and making a tea for uterine hemorrhaging. Some leaders have recommended you eat only one apple a year.
3. How can I justify referring some of my sickest patients to a counselor who has absolutely no medical training, possibly not even a high school education and maybe a week's crash course somewhere. There's no gold standard

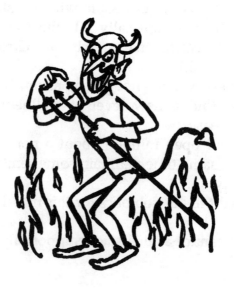

As with every new and controversial endeavor, you want to play the devil's advocate and look objectively at both sides (yin and yang).

by which we can measure competency in macrobiotic diagnosis and counseling. If you want to be safe you'd go to Michio Kushi in Becket Massachusetts. But I've taken care of patients who went there and were failures and eventually flew to Syracuse for treatment instead. I'm not knocking them. I'm sure they have healed failures of mine. I'm pointing out legitimate problems. I would like to see macrobiotics attain enough credibility that an institute such as Mr. Kushi's reaches a level of acceptance by the medical profession. This would entail a standard of excellence that we could count on as in any other medical specialty. This can only happen, as I see it, through scientific study.

Happily, as I see more and more people from around the country, I keep learning of more and more wonderful counselors that have helped them. They send me a referral letter or a copy of the recommendations they have made for my patient. This tells me they are proud enough of their work to become a member of our medical team.

Now this will make many people in macrobiotics very angry for just as in medicine, there are people who feel you must be all or nothing. They arrogantly feel you should be a total devotee of macrobiotics in every phase of your life. They dislike the idea of their diet being used for its own sake and even prophesied that it won't work without the whole philosophy. The problem is just as with yin and yang, nothing is absolute. And by the way, no two books can ever agree on that! Something as fundamental as what is yin and what is yang is fraught with controversy. Even Ohsawa called things yin in the seventies that years earlier he himself had called yang. And did you ever see what chaos results when you have a roomful of certified macro counselors discussing yin and yang? So don't feel bad if it confuses you.

Isn't it ironic—all we ever wanted was health. When medicine couldn't give it to us, we found answers in ecology. Then doctors and insurance companies got nasty because we were forced to look for wellness outside of their system. They wanted us to get well through their system of drugs and surgery.

Now we've found another aid, macrobiotics, and we'll probably have more people angry with us for not totally embracing their system. When will the world recognize biochemical individuality and allow us to freely pick and choose (while monitoring our bodies' responses) the best of all worlds for ourselves!

Since I wear three hats (conventional medicine, environmental medicine and macrobiotics), let's look at some of the most salient difficulties with macrobiotic philosophy.

1. It has many contradictions. They even have experts arguing whether a new food is yin or yang.
2. They reversed the Chinese definition of yin and yang, which adds to the confusion. Fortunately descriptive terms, expansive and contractive have supplemented.
3. Alkaline and acid do not directly apply to yin and yang. Furthermore, many sources disagree as to which foods fall into which categories. Even within the same work there are contradictions. For example, Aihara's classic **Acid and Alkaline** classifies azuki and tofu as yin acid forming (pg 90), but alkaline forming (pg. 38, 39); confusing for the neophyte. A clearer treatise of these issues is needed if macro is to grow into a self-help discipline as it espouses.

4. It gets too confusing as one is taught that processes of food preparation can alter the yin or yang properties of food.
5. After reading over two dozen macrobiotics works, there are many unanswered questions and no recognized authority to consult. Who can we ask?

On the other hand, there are many extremely helpful ideas that emerge from these works. So where do we go from here?

The discipline of macrobiotics is so comprehensive that many books must be consulted. A major text is in need, where important facts are collated. For example:

Did You Know?

That Wakame seaweed has more B12 than beef or pork?

That Kombu has twice as much B12 as eggs?

That broccoli, Brussels sprouts, collard greens, mustard greens and parsley have more vitamin C than oranges?

That millet has almost twice the iron as beef?

That kale has twice as much calcium as milk?

That ume plums have more calcium, iron, and phosphorus than apples, strawberries, or peaches?

That ume plums are excellent alkalinizers as well as being neutralizers of toxins and lactic acid (they work best for yin (sweets/alcohol) hangovers, while apple cider/kuzu or scallion/miso soup works better for yang (meat/salt) hangovers. Umeboshi is 20% salt, so limit to one a day.

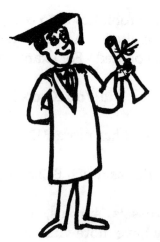

How does one know a counselor is good? There is no medically or even state recognized study program with certification. It takes the Chinese years to learn oriental diagnosis, but westerners can take 1-6 weeks of a course and call themselves counselors. There does not appear to be a governing/regulatory board.

That miso, tamari, and gomashio also help to neutralize symptoms from excessive smoke exposure? The first two are 13-18% salt so limit them, especially when in the healing mode.

That if you are caught out eating fish without any daikon or ume, you could order horseradish along with it?

That miso soup with scallion or barley are good to reduce the symptoms from meat?

That grated daikon and ginger help mobilize sticky mucous?

That cravings for coffee, beer, or cigarettes (bitter) can be helped by increasing your (bitter) greens (dandelion, etc.)?

That sweet cravings can be overcome with sweet grains and vegetables like sweet rice or your squash soup?

That too much sour can be counteracted by pungent (ginger)?

That sour counters pungent (ginger)
That bitter counters salty
That pungent counters bitter (greens)
That salty counters sweet
That sweet counters sour, etc.?

That one tbs. sesame seeds has more calcium than one cup of milk?

That millet, chickpeas, or lentils have more iron than beef liver?

So why are vitamin levels needed if this diet is so healthy?

Because with a diet of predominantly cooked foods, there can be a shortage of vitamins that are destroyed by heat, like B or C. And the work of detox depletes nutrients.

Rationale for Remedies

What factors contribute the worst to acidity?

1. Poor **nutritional status** from depleted soils, non-organic foods, processed foods and poor eating habits all stress the chemistry and push it to find compensatory routes.
2. An overloaded chemical environment causes stress to the xenobiotic detoxication system, through the formation of free radicals, which are crazy unfocused electrons that destroy cell membranes and initiate disease, increase and add to the acidity and biochemical stress.
3. A poorly balance diet with emphasis on sweets and meats creates a high acid stress.
4. Unhealthy thoughts like anger, worry, jealousy, fear, hate, and resentment cause the release of brain neurotransmitters which in turn trigger the release of hormones and peptides that add to the acidity to be neutralized by the body. More importantly, these emotions indicate there is imbalance (they are a symptom) which needs to be addressed.

Why is Acidity Bad?

Increased acid is the antagonist to good health. The body must constantly work to keep it in check. Likewise, increased alkalinity could create uncontrolled cravings or an extreme feeling of unwellness until it is corrected.

Acidity pulls calcium from bones so that early dental and jaw bone disease results with infections, root canals and eventual false teeth. Acidity uses up magnesium so cardiac arrhythmia and neck and back muscle spasms occur more easily with seemingly minor triggers. Or other smooth muscles go into spasm easily resulting in diarrhea, migraine, or asthma.

Although few sources agree, a rough approximation of foods (and drink and chemicals) can be categorized as I have portrayed them in the diagram (p 275). By studying this and the many texts that go into greater detail, you can begin to appreciate how you can manipulate your body chemically with what you choose to eat. You are like a perpetual laboratory experiment. You can control your health, your moods, and your energy by just observing and listening to the feedback. Isn't it exciting?

Acid and Alkaline, Yin and Yang, Expansive and Contractive

In order to heal the quickest it seems logical to take as much extraneous work away from the body as possible. After all, when you have a fever and pneumonia you don't dig ditches, you go to bed.

Since the body works hard at keeping the pH or hydrogen ion content at 7.43, it seems logical to eat near this with 50:50 whole grains and veggies as opposed to two colas and a candy bar.

And so the pH or acid/alkaline content of foods has been determined. It has another benefit because it helps you determine what to take to balance a craving. For example, if you've had an ice cream and feel sleepy and moody, try some ume plums to alkalinize your system.

Yin and yang are part of the oriental philosophy of opposites. They apply to every force of life and help establish our concept of balance. Everything has some yin and some yang qualities. Nothing is totally one or the other. Furthermore, the yinness or yangness of something is relative to everything else. Nothing stands alone.

We have modern sayings that express the duality of life and remind us to always look for the balance ("Every cloud has a silver lining"). And one of the seven laws of the Order of the Universe according to macrobiotic philosophy is "That which has a beginning has an end." That might be analogous to "It's always darkest before the dawn".

When yin and yang are applied to food, however, the picture becomes complicated. Acid and alkaline content can be measured in a laboratory. Yin and yang cannot. Not only that but some people spend their lives arguing over what is yin or yang. To further complicate matters, what Mr. Ohsawa called yin in 1928, he called yang in his 1960 writings. Yin and yang are also relative. A chicken is yang compared with fish, but is yin compared with salt.

George Ohsawa's terms expansive and contractive seem to handle our needs better. Although there is no across the board correlation, in general foods that are acid are also yin or expansive. Likewise, foods that are alkaline are often contractive or yang. You will find many exceptions to these however.

In general, contractiveness has features of being low growing, slow growing, and hard, needing long cooking. Yang alkaline foods include Bancha tea, dandelion tea, lotus root, burdock root, sesame and soy sauce, miso, salt, and umeboshi. Yang acid-forming foods include grains, fish, fowl, beef and eggs.

Yang foods tend to warm the body. Too much yang leads to contractive symptoms and tightness such as arthritis, arteriosclerosis, compact tumors or cancers, aggression, inflexibility and arrogance. These can be modified to good qualities of moral strength.

Expansiveness represents features of high growing, quick growing, soft, growing in a warm climate, being watery and big, and requiring little or no cooking. Yin acid-forming substances include chemicals, medications, sugar, alcohol, some beans, oils and nuts.

The expansive foods tend to cool the body. The symptoms of over expansiveness can be chemical allergies, hyper-sensitivity, edema, leukemia, spaciness, confusion, and inability to concentrate (brain fog or toxic encephalopathy). These can be modified to bring out one's artistic and creative nature.

Isn't it interesting that this age old philosophy describes our 21st century disease of E.I. perfectly?

But should this all sound a bit confusing, remember there are no absolutes. Nothing is totally yin or yang. Everything is relative to other things. Nor are yin and yang good or bad. They are in fact complimentary.....the spice of life. In fact, we need both in order to sustain life.

287

Very roughly speaking, acid/alkaline, expansive/contractive and yin/yang could look somewhat like this:

Yin Acid	Expansive	Yin Alkaline
chemicals		wine, colas
drugs, medicines		lemon, yogurt, ginger
sugar, candy		coffee, mineral water
vinegar		raisins, bananas
whiskey, beer		shitake, cinnamon
olive oil, sesame oil		apple, cherries
almonds, tofu		cabbage, broccoli
chickpeas		pumpkin, onion
azuki		daikon, nori, hiziki

*** Center ***

macaroni		seeds, squash
oats		carrots,
barley		milk
rice, wheat		kuzu tea
white fish		burdock, kombu
fowl		millet
meat		lotus
tuna, salmon		dandelion, mu tea
eggs		gomashio, soy sauce
ginseng		wakame
		miso, ume, salt

Yang Acid	Contractive	Yang Alkaline

As you see, the more extreme foods are at the ends; as far from the center as possible. You can easily appreciate how a specified amount of a food could be therapeutic but why an excess would help to create further imbalance. Your best guide is to listen to your unmasked body.

288

Basically you want to do the majority of your eating near the center or fulcrum of the balance scale. But when imbalance occurs, you can see what remedy would most likely correct it or bring you closer to the center again.

Clearly, by beginning to understand the acid/alkali format, you can understand why certain remedies work. Just don't go out on the ends away from the fulcrum unless you are in great health or it's a time for a festival. The majority of the time you want to give your body the room it needs to heal.

Say you've overdosed on sweets, or you have a craving for chocolate? Miso soup or umeboshi (plums) may take care of that for you. I use mustard greens (because I loved bitter chocolate) in chickpea miso soup, some barley (for the calories and hunger), and sprinkle gomashio over the top (for the crunchies). You could dangle bittersweet chocolate under my nose and I have no craving. I know it sounds bizarre because when I first tested umeboshi (plums), for example, I was sure everyone who used them was nuts. But once you establish balance and see how soothing they feel, you will learn to listen to your body and correct its imbalances. Remember, a craving is merely a transient chemical imbalance and with thoughtless binges you over-correct and use up too much biochemical energy. Also, you will shortly have another craving because you have overshot the mark. Giving in to a craving means indulging in an extreme food that throws you past the fulcrum to the opposite end of the scale.

In essence, when you are balanced, you feel satiated and comfortable and are not driven to eat in excess. Right now Americans have such distorted taste buds and body feedback/recognition systems that they eat only for taste and mood.

Say you have diarrhea, a very yin (expansive) symptom —
you could turn it off with a seaweed soup with miso, or
kuzu/umeboshi/soy sauce/bancha tea. This also helps a
sweet craving. There is lots more about all this in **THE CURE
IS IN THE KITCHEN.**

Or say you overdosed on meat; grated daikon with a few
drops of soy sauce will bring you back to the center. Carrot
or apple juice can also do the trick.

So you logically ask, why don't I balance meat with wine?
And obviously many cultures do so and quite healthfully.
But then you are pushing the extremes of the balance beam—
something you want to save for when you are healthy. The
further from the fulcrum, the more biochemical energy that
will be needed to establish balance. And you're trying to
reserve all of your energy for healing at this point in time.

I did well for a long time on sugar, wine, cheese, and meat.
The body breakdown steadily progressed, but I was able to
keep up by increasing my drugs for pain and other
symptoms. Then when the systems finally collapsed, I had
multiple target organ involvement, and I had exhausted my
wad of medicines. That's the time that a massive diet and
lifestyle change (environmental controls, assess thoughts and
goals) becomes necessary. That's when a plethora of
nutritional deficiencies must be sought and corrected:
meticulous attention to diet, nutritional status, environment,
and the psyche is required.

In the preceding macrobiotic scheme, it looks as though milk
should be a great buffer, but too many people know it gives

them tremendous nasal congestion and diarrhea. Likewise, many Candida and mold sensitive people cannot eat ferments like miso until they have been on the restricted macro diet for a few months and leveled out to a less extreme plateau.

Now you can begin to see how futile most diets are in helping weight loss, because cravings are not neutralized. For example, high meat (acid, contractive) creates a craving for the opposite for balance, hence alcohol and sugar (expansive) and/or coffee (alkaline). And likewise those who eat a large amount of fruits (expansive, alkaline) in the name of dieting, foster balancing cravings of salty foods like chips and pizza (contractive), sweets (acid), and meat (contractive, acid). Now you can see also why diets that rely on one kind of food are destined to fail in the long run.

Hunger after a meal most likely indicates imbalance; for starters, often it's time to abandon supplements. Next hunger can signify the need for protein foods or broken grains. Perhaps assimilation is poor. You may have an enzyme lack or the leaky gut syndrome. Lack of joy may indicate rigidity of one cooking style, or too much cooked food in general. Raw foods posses a life force that is destroyed by cooking.

It also appears on the chart that a diet balanced in sugar, coffee, meat and salt should make one feel pretty good, and indeed there are many healthy people who eat just that way. So why is it that some of us do so much better with grains and greens? It seems that biochemical individuality reigns over everything including macrobiotics.

In the words of David Yarrow, "Health is balance, and sickness is imbalance". Our medicine is simply the way we live. The mind and body are complementary and form a

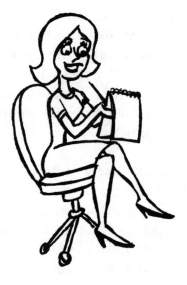

Even though they are not certified, there are several good counselors in our area. Since they don't send referral letters like physicians do, you'll need to send me an audio tape of your consultation if you want us to be part of your care.

unified whole. They are yin and yang. Problems in either will create distress and disorder in the opposite.

Nearly everyone with E.I. has a severe acid-alkaline imbalance. Not only are most too acidic, but their ability to neutralize and remove acid is severely disturbed and exhausted. Two primary alkalinizing minerals in the body are sodium and calcium. Today many people rely on heavy doses of salt and dairy to alkalinize the acid (or meats, sweets and processed foods). Many stones (and arteriosclerotic deposits) result from insoluble mineral salts condensing in the kidneys, gall bladder, (and blood vessels). Fresh vegetables (from sea and land) are the primary alkalinizing foods. Whole grains are next, with much individual variation. Thorough chewing alkalinizes whole grains. Kuzu-umeboshi tea can provide fast relief for many acid conditions from sour stomach to fatigue.

Mucous is a general term for the waste and debris in the system. Dairy, oils, sugar, and baked flour products are the primary offenders. This excess mucous can eventually be eliminated through the intestine with a macrobiotic diet of whole grains and vegetables. Onion, daikon, cruciferous vegetables (cabbage, cauliflower, broccoli, kale, collards, Brussels sprouts, etc.) garlic and barley are among the foods that can help in dissolving this material. Seaweeds are a vital source of precious balanced minerals to strengthen the body buffering fluids, white ginger, exercise and skin brushing help to stimulate the circulation.

For all its strangeness, inconsistencies and drawbacks, macrobiotics has the potential to turn around our present epidemic in disguise of subclinical malnutrition. It also has the potential to arrest and even reverse a vast amount of degenerative disease (which this subclinical malnutrition has contributed to). Macrobiotics also embraces the reality that we are a part of the macro and micro cosmos. When this is realized, it makes it difficult for an intelligent person to knowingly pollute his body with inferior food, pesticides, additives and drugs and to pollute his environment with acid rain, nuclear and chemical wastes. On the home front he will opt for a chemically less-contaminated lifestyle as well.

By checking for nutrient (vitamin, mineral, essential fatty acid, amino acid) balance, we hope to maximize wellness and further substantiate the benefits of macrobiotics. By documenting the discharge phenomenon (liver functions, monitoring depurated xenobiotics) we are trying to establish a scientific rationale for macrobiotics. Then, and only then can medical acceptance come about, which in turn should lead to wider acceptance and availability of wholesome foods on airlines and in restaurants. The global benefits are awesome.

Meanwhile, after 25 years of practicing medicine, I know of very few other modalities that are so simultaneously healing (against all odds) and inexpensive and available to everyone. It seems foolish to ignore it if you have been paddling upstream for too long in your quest for wellness. I have witnessed many heal the impossible.

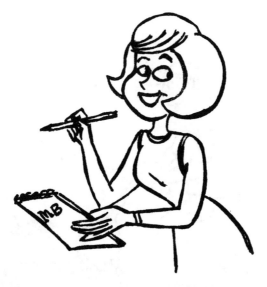

Don't forget to bring both questionnaires, filled out beforehand, to every visit. Otherwise, we'll have to spend time asking you all those background questions and won't have time for the actual consultation.

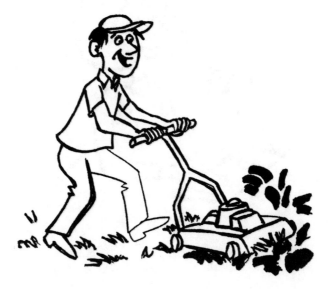

Most people have spouses who mow the lawn. My poor husband can usually find his wife grazing on the lawn instead. I eat most of my dandelions.

BIOCHEMICAL BLUNDERS:
THE INNOCENCE OF MEDICINE?

In the following table which compares the philosophy of conventional medicine with that of macrobiotics and environmental medicine, it can be seen how naive conventional medicine is. Is this true innocence or waiting for the impossible, yet eternal dream of double blind proof?

The FDA usually requires double blind proof which works for drugs and surgeries, but not lifestyle changes. With a new drug you give 100 people the real thing and 100 people a dummy capsule. The physician and patients are unaware of which anyone is receiving until the study is over (hence double blind). Or is it an intentional criteria to ensure that only drugs will be condoned? For as you will read in **WELLNESS AGAINST ALL ODDS**, once you start on the drug highway, you will inevitably require more (and hasten your deterioration).

It seems that the environmental approach is so logical that the only dissenters that will remain are those motivated by ego and money before health.

I don't mean to place blame anywhere, and certainly not with the overworked, over-harassed physician. The poor guy studied diligently and works his best to apply what he learned in medical school. Somewhere along the line in our training though, respect for biochemical individuality and ecologically sound lifestyles was lost. Instead, we capriciously pollute our food, air and water. And when this causes symptoms, we use drugs to suppress them.

Fortunately, environmental, nutritional, biochemical, and

toxicologic research has accumulated sufficient data to usher in a more responsible era. A renaissance in medicine is here.

View On:	As seen by Conventional Medicine:	Environmental Medicine and Macrobiotics:
Drugs	a necessary part of overcoming illness	rarely necessary if a healthy body is maintained with chemically clean air, food, and water
Illness	seen as bad, requiring drugs to suppress symptoms	seen as good; an opportunity to cleanse, identify and correct an imbalance
Environment	something to be manipulated, fought and changed to suit our whims	an irreplaceable resource to be appreciated and harmonized with
People	all the same	no two alike due to biochemical individuality
Medicine	cookbook style	individualized
Vitamins	not needed in general	crucial to replace through whole foods and/or supplements;
Nutrient deficiencies	deficiencies unlikely as "The diet gives you everything you need".	deficiencies due to processed foods and the current extra stress on detoxification systems

Processed Foods	many healthy people live on them	undesirable; studies show inferior nutrition
Diet	very little influence over medical conditions	a major determinant of health
Health	absence of diagnosable disease	looking, feeling and and performing great
Diagnosis of disease	mostly through documentation of abnormal blood test, cultures, physical abnormality, or X-ray	consists of any symptoms that inhibit maximum wellness and perform-ance
Masking	non-existent	once you're eating well, your body alarms ring (symptoms) when you eat something that it doesn't like or need until it becomes adapted; then the alarm is muted or masked
Adaptation	inconsequential	the price to be paid for chronic adaptation is chronic disease
Cravings	silly, meaningless whimsical, lack of will-power	an important symptom of biochemical imbalance
Control of health	lies with the physician	lies with the individual; physician is the consultant

Treatment	all people with the same disease should have the same treatment	treatment is individual, no two people are alike
Minor Complaints	usually due to hypochondriasis, stress or depression	symptom of biochemical imbalance; an early warning of more severe disease to come
Aging	unchangeable	some genetic control but also the total accumulation of free radical destruction mediated by chronic overcompensation and adaptation to environmental over-load
Individual Person	a clone of everyone else	each one biochemically unique: one man's meat is another man's poison or to put it macro-biotically, one man's weeds are another man's dinner
Chronic degenerative disease	to be expected and accepted; unavoidable	having an environmental trigger, abnormal and controllable
Relation of man's health to environment	little bearing	a major factor, that cannot be ignored if wellness is to be attained

The naiveté of medicine when it comes to nutritional matters is startling in view of its fantastic accomplishments in other areas.

Take these four simple examples:

1. **The calcium craze.** Doctors have recommended everything from antacids to bone meal, without a thought of the need to balance this calcium carefully with other nutrients. And cognizance for the causes is not appreciated. If one reads the biochemistry literature, it's quite apparent that processed foods are high in phosphates. Phosphates in turn inhibit the absorption of calcium.

   Also, a high acid diet (processed foods, sweets, carbonated drinks, meats) uses up calcium as a buffer, stealing it from the bone. And if zinc, copper magnesium, boron, manganese and other trace elements are deficient, as they commonly are due to processed foods and devitalized soils, then calcium cannot be incorporated into bone. As far as supplementation goes, hypochlorhydria (low stomach acid) and antacids inhibit absorption and many recommended forms of calcium have very poor absorption to begin with. And again, if the status of the accessory minerals are not known and adjusted, there will be limited incorporation of the calcium into bone, regardless of amount and form recommended.

2. **The cholesterol controversy.** Doctors recommend diets of plastic foods (artificial eggs, butters, sausages), and dangerous transfatty acids (margarine, processed foods, polyunsaturated vegetable oils) that promote free radical damage (degenerative disease, allergies, cancer). When that fails, they prescribe cholesterol-lowering drugs that also inhibit the uptake of important nutrients and potentiate cancer. Don't forget, when you're nutrient

depleted, the last thing you want is another drug that further depletes more nutrients.

3. **Alzheimer's disease.** Billions of dollars are spent yearly on sustaining victims of this disease. But where is the education of doctors and the public to reduce their intake of aluminum? How many people use aluminum cookware and cans, antacids, douches, deodorants and foods? Aluminum is in many processed foods, salt, baking powder, cheeses, beer, and as an anti-caking agent in flour products, etc. Plus undetected calcium, zinc or magnesium deficiencies allow aluminum to be deposited more easily in the brain.

4. **Unrecognized zinc deficiency.** The literature supports the presence of a silent epidemic of zinc deficiency. Yet an RBC (red blood cell) zinc is not part of a routine chemical profile. No foods are fortified with zinc (except a few baby formulas). And yet it's crucial in every metabolic pathway of the body and a deficiency can help promote cancer, AIDS, chemical intolerance, other nutritional deficiencies and more.

All of these medical blunders and more are described in more detail in either **TIRED OR TOXIC?, WELLNESS AGAINST ALL ODDS,** or **DEPRESSION CURED AT LAST!** We are in essence going out of our way to become unhealthy quicker. Take one example. A gal is magnesium deficient from years of sweets. Her doctor prescribes calcium to prevent osteoporosis without assessing her mineral status (the tests are described in **TIRED OR TOXIC?**). This competes with magnesium to further lower it. Meanwhile she takes up jogging, sweats out more magnesium and ends up with terrible muscle spasms and pain (from magnesium

302

deficiency) after some back trauma. Or she can have a fatal cardiac arrhythmia from the magnesium deficiency.

Those were just four simple examples of current medical problems that could be corrected by just avoiding a processed foods diet. And left unchecked, each one can cause severely debilitating chronic symptoms and one symptom can be fatal. How very cost effective it would be to educate people about the value of eating whole foods and checking a simple RBC zinc blood test and the magnesium loading test. But first the medical school curriculum must teach the biochemistry of nutrition and environmental medicine.

There is already a plethora of evidence. On one hand we have a silent epidemic of malnutrition that contributes to chronic degenerative illness. And on the other, we have a diet of whole foods with a great track record for healing the impossible. What are we waiting for?

We've distorted our precious feedback system by eating processed foods. We crave sweets, fats, salts, and drinks. We overwork the gastrointestinal tract, liver and kidneys as well as plug arteries and put on unwanted weight.

Worst of all, we suffer anger, jealousy, depression, aggression, and self-pity. Don't forget, if you're standing on one leg, it's easier to knock you over. Well, if you're not playing with a full deck of nutrients, it's easier to create disease in you. And disease is not limited to physical symptoms. When you're not biochemically balanced, it's easy for seemingly inconsequential triggers to throw you into a rage. Remember just a zinc deficiency alone can affect a number of brain chemicals and neurotransmitters that control happy moods and stability. Mood swings, unhappiness and lack of enthusiasm are symptoms.

Likewise, faulty neurotransmitters (the brain's "happy hormones") that result can further distort the system. This in turn can lead to increased vulnerability, reactions, and symptoms, many of which are cerebral. It's a vicious cycle or a downward spiral that can lead to poor learning ability, poor social skills, poor school and work performances, delinquency and crime. The handwriting is on the wall.

Likewise, bad chemistry coupled with bad food and environment accelerates aging. In biochemical terms, aging is nothing more than free radical attack on cell membranes resulting in loss of flexibility. Inflexible cell membranes can lead to swelling or heart problems, arteriosclerosis, senility and organ damage. The body becomes inflexible as does the mind. In fact, that may be the problem with our detractors.

A 1987 survey of 11,000 people by the National Cancer Institute in Washington concluded that 80% of the 11,000 people interviewed never ate whole grains. Other than potatoes and salad, 49% never ate vegetables. Another 40% never had a daily fruit. But 40% had daily nitrate-containing bacon or luncheon meat.

In the same year, the director of the division of Cancer Prevention and Control for NCI stated at a Florida conference, "There is now general scientific evidence that about 80% of cancer cases appear to be linked to the way people live their lives. The role of diet in the cause and prevention of cancer is particularly important". Too bad it took until 1987 to figure this out. Others have known it for decades.

304

The bottom line is that environmental medicine coupled with macrobiotics is light years ahead of conventional medicine in terms of chronic disease. On the other hand, conventional medicine cannot be surpassed in its handle on acute disease. It's time for a marriage of the two. The stormy courtship is over.

HOW MUCH DOES DIET AFFECT HEALTH?

For a long time, the diet-health connection was limited to alcohol causing cirrhosis (liver damage), sugars exacerbating diabetes, and fats contributing to arteriosclerosis and coronary artery disease.

Thanks to the research efforts of hundreds of epidemiologists and other scientists, it is now a well-substantiated fact that dietary fat also has an enormous bearing on the development of prostate cancer, breast cancer, and every other cancer. On the flip side, the correct fats are essential for life and optimum body function. Lack of proper fats causes disease.

In recent years, scientists have dissected the very chemicals in foods that are part of the macrobiotic diet. They want to discover, re-synthesize, and sell the healing ingredients. They have found that such phyto (plant) - chemicals can not only stop the development of cancer, but can turn it off once it has begun. One example is sulforaphane in broccoli. But instead of advising a helping of one of the cruciferous vegetables each day, they are trying to make it into a pill. It will cost much more than just eating well, and (since you cannot one-up God) will not be as effective. Some phytochemicals are already on the market, substantiating this prediction.

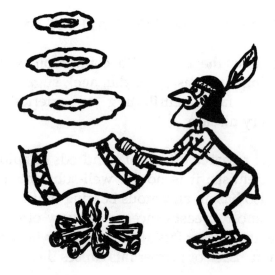

Communication is the key. We've racked up enough successes; now we need to medically document it and publish it. We need your help in keeping us posted on your progress. Blood tests are useful to document discharge and improvement in nutrient levels.

WHERE DO I GO FROM HERE?

If you are serious about seeing what the macrobiotic diet, which has clearly healed the impossible, can do for you, next read **THE CURE IS IN THE KITCHEN.** If you are not ready to take the plunge, ease into a transition diet by using **MACRO MELLOW.** If you are quite sick, **WELLNESS AGAINST ALL ODDS** is a must, followed by **TIRED OR TOXIC?,** then **DEPRESSION CURED AT LAST!** Don't let the last title fool you. It is not totally limited to depression, but covers the blueprint for every illness.

If you have a doctor whom you would like to interest in this, give him first **THE SCIENTIFIC BASIS FOR SELECTED ENVIRONMENTAL MEDICINE TECHNIQUES,** then **TIRED OR TOXIC?** If he gets hooked, **"WELLNESS"** followed by **"DEPRESSION"** will keep him hooked and eager to learn more. Then you will have a great ally on your side, as it is worth the effort. If you've never read **THE E.I. SYNDROME, REVISED,** you'll need to round out your medical education by including that.

For this is the first medical specialty where the patient must become an expert. There are 2 basic ways to approach illness: drugs or diet. If you choose the diet route, you (1) save money, (2) can actually heal, rather than merely masking symptoms with drugs, (3) you stop the cycle of one disease blossoming into many others, (4) and you learn how to keep yourself healthy ever after. The price you pay is to educate yourself. And you have already made a huge step in that direction, since you now know that YOU ARE WHAT YOU ATE.

NOTE FROM THE DOCTOR

As a specialist in environmental medicine who is on the leading edge (which also means the firing line!), I am grateful for all that my illness has taught me, and for all that my patients have taught me. I am grateful for all the discoveries of biochemists and toxicologists around the world (however incredibly ignored they may be by the medical profession), and I am grateful for macrobiotics and the people who brought it to us. In order to return that gratitude, I think macrobiotics deserves more careful study and documentation so that we may give a gift in return; widespread acceptance and appreciation of its principles. For even if you find that you graduate to a carnivore or live food diet, the principles you learned (preparation of whole grains, molybdenum - rich beans, a huge variety of vegetables, mineral - rich sea vegetables, etc.) will serve you well regardless of path.

Clearly, you now can appreciate more than ever that you have great control through food over your health and your moods. Truly, **YOU ARE WHAT YOU ATE.**

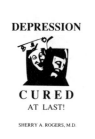

DEPRESSION

CURED
AT LAST!

SHERRY A. ROGERS, M.D.

DEPRESSION CURED AT LAST! Just when you think all has been accomplished, along comes the most important book of all. Unique in many ways, (1) it is written for the lay person and the physician, and is appropriate as a medical school text book. In fact, it should be required reading for all physicians regardless of specialty.

(2) It shows that it borders on malpractice to treat depression as a Prozac deficiency, to drug cardiology patients, or any other medical/psychiatric problem without first ruling out proven causes.

With over a 700 pages and 1,000 complete references it covers the environmental, nutritional and metabolic causes of all disease. It covers leaky gut syndrome, intestinal dysbiosis, hormone deficiencies, hidden sensitivities to foods, molds, and chemicals, dysfunctional detoxication, heavy metal and pesticide poisonings, xenobiotic accumulations, and much, much more.

It is the best blue-print for figuring out what is wrong and how to fix it once and for all. If no one knows what is wrong with you, you need this book. If they know but say there is no cure, you need this book. If they say you need medications to control your symptoms indefinitely, you need this book.

It is inconceivable that there is anyone who would not benefit from this book as it surely leaves drug-oriented medicine in the dust of the 20th century. And it does so by using the only disease that by definition sports a lack of hope. We chose this disease, depression, as a prototype to be sure to drive home the message that just when you least expect it, there is always **hope**.

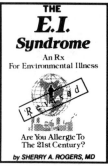

THE E.I.
Syndrome
An Rx
For Environmental Illness

Are You Allergic To
The 21st Century?

by SHERRY A. ROGERS, MD

THE E.I. SYNDROME, REVISED is a 635 page book that is necessary for people with environmental illness. It explains chemical, food, mold, and Candida sensitivities, nutritional deficiencies, testing methods and how to do the various environmental controls and diets in order to get well.

Many docs buy these by the hundreds and make them mandatory reading for patients, as it contains many pearls about getting well that are not found anywhere else. In this way it increases the fun of practicing medicine because patients are on a higher educational level and office time is more productive for more sophisticated levels of wellness. It covers hundreds of facts that make the difference between E.I. victims versus E.I. conquerors. It helps patients become active partners in their care while avoiding doctor burn-out. It covers the gamut of the diagnosis and treatment of environmentally induced symptoms.

Because the physician author was a severe universal reactor who has recovered, this book contains mountains of clues to wellness. As a result many have written that they healed themselves by reading this book. This is in spite of the fact, that no consulted physicians were able to diagnose or effectively treat them. If you are not sure what causes your symptoms, this is a great start.

Many veteran sufferers have written that they had read many books on aspects of allergy, chronic Candidiasis and chemical sensitivity and thought that they knew it all. Yet they wrote that what they learned in THE E.I. SYNDROME REVISED enabled them to reach that last pinnacle of wellness.

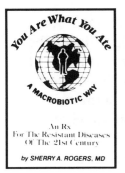

An Rx
For The Resistant Diseases
Of The 21st Century

by SHERRY A. ROGERS, MD

YOU ARE WHAT YOU ATE. This book is dispensable as a primer and introduction to the macrobiotic diet. The macrobiotic diet is the specialized diet with which many have healed the impossible, including end stage metastatic cancers. This is after medicine had given up on them and they had been given only months or weeks to live. Yes, they have rallied after surgery, chemotherapy and radiation had failed. Life was seemingly, hopelessly over.

Understandably, this diet has also enabled many chemically sensitive universal reactors, and highly allergic and even "undiagnosable people" to heal. It has also enabled those to heal that have "wastebasket" diagnostic labels such as chronic fatigue, fibromyalgia, MS, rheumatoid arthritis, depression, chronic infections, colitis, asthma, migraines, lupus, chronic Candidiasis, and much more.

Although there are many books on macrobiotics, this is one that takes the special needs of the allergic person and those with multiple food and chemical sensitivities as well as chronic Candidiasis into account. It provides details and case histories that the person new to macrobiotics needs before he embarks on the strict healing phase as described in **THE CURE IS IN THE KITCHEN.**

Even people who have done the macrobiotic diet for a while will find reasons why they have failed and tips to improve their success. When a diet such as this has allowed many to heal their cancers, any other condition "should be a piece of cake".

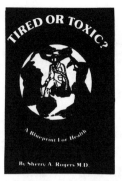

TIRED OR TOXIC? is a 400 page book, and the first book that describes the mechanism, diagnosis and treatment of chemical sensitivity, complete with scientific references. It is written for the layman and physician alike and explains the many vitamin, mineral, essential fatty acid and amino acid analyses that may help people detoxify everyday chemicals more efficiently and hence get rid of baffling symptoms.

It is the first book written for laymen and physicians to describe xenobiotic detoxication, the process that allows all healing to occur. You have heard of the cardiovascular system, you have heard of the respiratory system, the gastrointestinal system, and the immune system. But most have never heard of the chemical detoxification system that is the determinant of whether we have chemical sensitivity, cancer, and in fact every disease.

This program shows how to diagnose and treat many resistant everyday symptoms and use molecular medicine techniques. It also gives the biochemical mechanisms in easily understood form, of how Candida creates such a diversity of symptoms and how the macrobiotic diet heals "incurable" end stage metastatic cancers. It is a great book for the physician you are trying to win over, and will show you how chemical sensitivity masquerades as common symptoms. It then explores the many causes and cures of chemical sensitivity, chronic Candidiasis, and other "impossible to heal" medical labels.

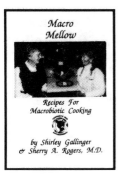

Macro Mellow

Recipes For Macrobiotic Cooking

by Shirley Gallinger & Sherry A. Rogers, M.D.

MACRO MELLOW is a book designed for 4 types of people: (1) For the person who doesn't know a thing about macrobiotics, but just plain wants to feel better, in spite of the 21st century. (2) It solves the high cholesterol/triglycerides problem without drugs and is the preferred diet for heart disease patients. (3) It is the perfect transition diet for those not ready for macro, but needing to get out of the chronic illness rut. (4) It spells out how to feed the rest of the family who hates macro, while another family member must eat it in order to clear their "incurable" symptoms.

It shows how to convert the "grains, greens, and beans" strict macro food into delicious "American-looking" food that the kids will eat. This saves the cook from making double meals while one person heals. The delicious low-fat whole food meals designed by Shirley Gallinger, a veteran nurse who has worked with Dr. Rogers for nearly two decades, use macro ingredients without the rest of the family even knowing. It is the first book to dove-tail creative meal planning, menus, recipes and even gardening so the cook isn't driven crazy.

Most likely your kitchen contains a plethora of cookbooks. But you owe it to yourself and your family to learn how to incorporate healing whole foods, low in fat and high in phyto-nutrients into their diets. Who you have planning and cooking your meals has been proven to be as important if not more important than who you have chosen for your doctor. Medical research has proven the power of whole food diets to heal where high tech medicines and surgery have failed.

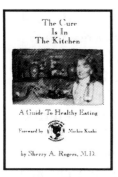

THE CURE IS IN THE KITCHEN is the next book you should read after YOU ARE WHAT YOU ATE. It is the first book to ever spell out in detail what all those people ate day to day who cleared their incurable diseases, MS, rheumatoid arthritis, fibromyalgia, lupus, chronic fatigue, colitis, asthma, migraines, depression, hypertension, heart disease, angina, undiagnosable symptoms, and relentless chemical, food, Candida, and electromagnetic sensitivities, as well as terminal cancers.

Dr. Rogers flew to Boston each month to work side by side with Mr. Michio Kushi, as he counseled people at the end of their medical ropes. As their remarkable case histories will show you, nothing is hopeless. Many of these people had failed to improve with surgery, chemotherapy and radiation. Instead their metastases continued to spread. It was only when they were sent home to die within a few weeks, that they turned to the diet.

Medical studies confirmed that this diet has more than tripled the survival from cancers. And the beauty of this diet is that you use God-given whole foods to coax the body into the healing mode. It does not rely on prescription drugs, but allows the individual to heal himself at home.

If you cannot afford a $500 consultation, and you choose not to accept your death sentence or medication sentence, why not learn first hand what these people did and how you, too, may improve your health and heal the impossible.

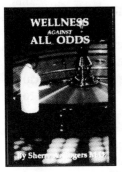

WELLNESS AGAINST ALL ODDS is the 6th and most revolutionary book by Sherry A. Rogers, M.D. It contains the ultimate healing plan that people have successfully used to beat cancer when they were given 2 weeks, some even 2 days to live by some of the top medical centers. These people had exhausted all that medicine has to offer, including surgery, chemotherapy, radiation and bone marrow transplants. Some had even been macrobiotic failures. And one of the most unbelievable things is that the plan costs practically nothing to implement and most of it can be done at home with non-prescription items.

Of course, in keeping with the other works and going far beyond, this contains the mechanisms of how these principles heal and is complete with all the scientific references for physicians.

Did you know, for example, that there are vitamins that actually cure some cancers, and over 50 papers in the best medical journals to prove it? Likewise, did you know that there are non-prescription enzymes that dissolve cancer, arteriosclerotic plaque, and auto-antibodies like lupus and rheumatoid? Did you know that there is a simple inexpensive, but highly effective way to detoxify the body at home to stop the toxic side effects of chemotherapy within minutes? Did you know that this procedure can also reduce chemical sensitivity reactions (from accidental chemical exposures) from 4 days to 20 minutes? Did you know that there are many hidden causes for "undiagnosable" symptoms that are never looked for, because it is easier and quicker to prescribe a pill than find (and fix) the causes?

The fact is that when you get the body healthy enough, it can heal anything. You do not have to die from labelitis. It no longer matters what your label is, from chronic Candida, fatigue, or MS to chemical sensitivity, an undiagnosable condition, or the worst cancer with only days to survive. If you have been told there is nothing more that can be done for you, you have the option of kicking death in the teeth and healing the impossible. Are you game?

The
Scientific Basis
for
Selected
Environmental
Medicine
Techniques

by

Sherry A. Rogers, M.D.

THE SCIENTIFIC BASIS FOR SELECTED ENVIRONMENTAL MEDICINE TECHNIQUES contains the scientific evidence and references for the techniques of environmental medicine. It is designed with the patient in mind who is being denied medical payments by insurance companies that refuse to acknowledge environmental medicine.

With this guide a patient may choose to represent himself in small claims court and quote from the book showing, for example, that the **JOURNAL OF THE AMERICAN MEDICAL ASSOCIATION** states that "titration provides a useful and effective measure of patient sensitivity", and that a U.S. Government agency states that "an exposure history should be taken for every patient". Failure to do so can lead to an inappropriate diagnosis and treatment.

It has sections showing medical references of how finding hidden vitamin deficiencies have, for example, enabled people to heal carpal tunnel syndrome without surgery, or heal life threatening steroid-resistant vasculitis, or stop seizures, or migraines, or learning disabilities.

This book is designed for patients who choose to find the causes of their illnesses rather than merely mask their symptoms with drugs for the rest of their lives. It is also for those who have been unfairly denied insurance coverage. And it is the ideal book with which to educate your PTA, attorney, insurance company, or physicians who still doubt your sanity.

In this era many HMO's tell people what diseases they can have, how long they can have them, and what treatments they can have. And all diseases seem to be deficiencies of drugs, for that is how they are all treated. It is as though arthritis were an Advil deficiency. This book arms you with the ammunition to defend your right to find the causes and get rid of symptoms and drugs.

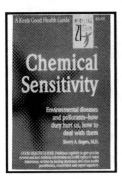

CHEMICAL SENSITIVITY. This 48 page booklet is the most concise referenced booklet on chemical sensitivity. It is for the person wanting to learn about it but who is leery of tackling a big book. It is ideal for teaching your physician or convincing your insurance company, as it is fully referenced. And it is a good reference for the veteran who wants a quick concise review.

Most people have difficulty envisioning chemical sensitivity as a potential cause of everyday maladies. But the fact is that a lack of knowledge of the mechanism of chemical sensitivity can be the solo reason that holds many back from ever healing completely. Some will never get truly well simply because they do not comprehend the tremendous role chemical sensitivity plays. For failure to address the role that chemical sensitivity plays in every disease has been pivotal in failure to get well. The principles of environmental controls are of especially vital importance for cancer victims.

If you are not completely well, you need to read this book. If you have been sentenced to a life-time of drugs, whether it be for high blood pressure, high cholesterol, angina, arrhythmia, asthma, eczema, sinusitis, colitis, learning disabilities, or cancer, you need this book. It matters not what your label is. What matters is whether chemical sensitivity is a factor that no one has explored that is keeping you from getting well. Most probably it is, and this is an inexpensive way to start you on the path toward drug-free wellness.

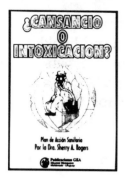

Cansancio o Intoxicacion?

El lego informado reconoce que a medida que el mundo se vuelve más tecnológico, el hombre pierde proporcionalmente más control sobre su vida. Este libro le permitirá recuperar el control de su salud, ofreciéndole mayor capacidad para formar equipo con su medico para diagnosticar y tratar su condición.

Esta información es vitalmente importante ahora ya que a todos toca con cualquier síntoma tal como la sensibilidad química, alto colesterol, fatiga crónica, complejo relacionado a Cándida, depresion, Alzheimer, hipertensión, diabetes, enfermedad cardíaca, osteoporosis y más.

Dra. Rogers se encuentra en la avanazada de la educación pública sobre los efectos del medio ambiente en el individuo.

Otros libros escritos por Dra. Rogers que tienen que ver con prevenir enfermedades y restablecer la salud son **Eres lo que Has Comido, El Síndrome de E.A., y La Cura Se Encuentra En La Cocina:** La Fase Curativa Estricta de la Dieta Macrobiotica.

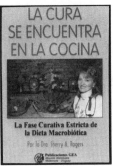

La Cura Se Encuentra En La Cocina

Este libro explora la relación entre dieta, medio ambiente, salud, y enfermedad y explica como la dieta macrobiótica, basada en cereales integrales, porotos y sus productos y otros alimentos naturales integrales puede prevenir enfermedades y restablecer la salud.

Nos explica cómo una dieta muy artificial contribuye a una variedad de problemas de salud y cómo ciertos aspectos de la vida moderna también nos pueden debilitar.

Un programa macrobiótico consiste de dos fases; pasar gradualmente a una dieta macrobótica o ponerse en una fase curativa estricta de carácter temporario. El objectivo de la fase curativa de esta dieta es aclarar una condición en particular. Es necesariamente, muy estricta e individualizada, y por eso razón, la persona debe consultar un doctor entrenado en la macrobiótica.

Otros libros escritos por Dra. Rogers que tienen que ver con prevenir enfermedades y restablecer la salud son **Cansancio o Intoxicación?, Eres lo que Has Comido,** y **El Síndrome de E.A.**

TOTAL HEALTH IN TODAY'S WORLD

This referenced monthly **newsletter** will keep you up to date on new findings. Since Dr. Rogers is constantly researching, lecturing around the globe, maintaining a private practice, doing television and radio shows, writing for health magazines and physicians, and has published 17 scientific papers and 9 books in 10 years, she is peddling as fast as she can.

There is literally an avalanche of new information, but we don't want you to have to wait for a new book on the subject to learn about it. We want that practical and useful instruction in your hands this month.

Furthermore, the field of environmental medicine, because it is so all-encompassing, can be overwhelming at times. So in addition to bringing you the new, we also focus on the perspective and when to resort to the basics.

In this era, because we cannot get the information out to you fast enough, we use the newsletter as our communication link. It will teach you useful facts years before they will be presented elsewhere, and it is practical and action-oriented. For pennies a day, you really cannot afford to be without it.

ENVIRONMENTAL MEDICINE VIDEO

On this 16 minute VHS video, Dr. Sherry Rogers teaches the basic principles of environmental medicine and chemical sensitivity. As you begin to learn how to diagnose and treat using environmental medicine techniques, it opens up a whole new world of options for getting well, regardless of diagnosis.

Also there are actual case presentations who will explain aspects of their emergence from E.I. (environmental illness) victims to E.I. conquerors. Each of them as well as Dr. Rogers herself were highly chemically sensitive and learned how to heal. This shows newly diagnosed people that there is hope.

This is a great video for the PTA, church groups, work groups, and special disease support groups to whom you want to introduce the concept of chemical sensitivity.

MOLD PLATES

Since mold is a common, yet remedial cause of symptoms, you first need to know if you have too much. By exposing special petri dishes (or mold plates) in your bedroom, family room, and office, you have effectively assessed your 24 hour mold environment.

Each plate comes with directions for exposure and a return mailer. In 6-9 weeks after the slow-growing fungi have appeared for identification, the report will be mailed to you detailing all of the specific molds and how many molds are present. We purposely take as long as we need, since we wait for the last molds to grow out before completing the report. We do not want to neglect the "slow growing" molds like other labs do, often sending reports back within days of receiving the plates. You will need to order one plate for each room you want to assess at home or work.

If you do not know how moldy your environment is, you may erroneously be attributing symptoms to chemical or food sensitivities. It is always best to meet the enemy head on in order to identify the cause of the problem and solve it, once and for all.

FORMALDEHYDE SPOT TEST KIT

The Formaldehyde Spot Test is a colorimetric test to determine whether you have too many objects in your home or office environments that outgas formaldehyde. Formaldehyde sensitivity can begin in anyone at any time. It masquerades as a variety of undiagnosable symptoms. And if you do not have the correct diagnosis, then medications will most likely be resorted to for symptom control. But adding another chemical to the body of one who is already over-burdened by his attempts at chemical detoxification, can make the sick get sicker, quicker.

One kit tests over a hundred objects in your environment. You merely put a drop of the solution on papers, furnishings, carpet, mattresses, wallboard, clothes, textiles, draperies, or just sitting on the glass slide to measure ambient air. If it turns dark purple, it has picked up over 10 ppm (parts per million) of formaldehyde and is an object that is contributing to your total load. That amount of formaldehyde emission is putting a strain on the body's detoxification pathways. And if they are strained, then the ability to detoxify everyday chemicals that can cause the genetic changes that initiate cancer and other diseases, can occur more readily.

Once you know which objects are contributing to your total load, you are better equipped to make some intelligent choices about your environment. And when you know what the worst culprits are, it spares you the aggravation of getting rid of items that are too dear, too costly, or too difficult to remove. Even for general health reasons, it is preferable to know which objects may be contributing to current or future ill-health. For formaldehyde sensitivity can begin at any time and manifest as merely mood swings, depression, migraines, or asthma, arthritis, brain fog, eye irritation, cough, nasal congestion, weakened immune system, the beginning of multiple new allergies, fatigue, fibromyalgia, and much more.

As well, objects that are outgassing too much formaldehyde are often outgassing other xenobiotics (foreign chemicals). So by knowing which ones to get rid of, you will often be simultaneously lowering your load to toluene, xylene, benzene, and other common household and office chemicals which are disease-promoting.

PHYSICIAN SLIDE SHOW

This 35 mm presentation contains 56 slides plus the script, which the physician can read or easily memorize. It is a great way for him to introduce to colleagues his incorporation of environmental medicine techniques into his practice. He can present this lecture as "The Biochemistry of Chemical Sensitivity" to other physicians at the hospital to further substantiate his rapidly expanding and firm foundation of knowledge in the field of environmental medicine.

Instructions then tell how with minor reorganization, he can use the same lecture retitled "Are You Tired or Toxic?" to present to lay groups like church groups, the PTA, and other special interest support groups to advertise his expertise in this area. As time rolls on he can add slides of his own such as case examples and new information as his audiences grow in sophistication.

It is meant to simultaneously instruct as well as build his credibility and practice. And you actually learn yourself as you rehearse it. He can also deflect the cost of renting an auditorium by selling the companion books (TIRED OR TOXIC?, CHEMICAL SENSITIVITY, and DEPRESSION CURED AT LAST!) after the talk (available at 40% discount in quantities of 40 or more). Subsequently, as people learn more about the environmental medicine approach to solve their medical problems, they progressively appreciate the limitations of the drug-oriented approach and find less use for it.

Remember, you can be a terrific physician, but if no one knows of your expertise or the rationale for referring recalcitrant patients to you, your talent may lay dormant and wasted. Happily, you will find that every time you present your lecture, many in the audience will benefit from being introduced to these revolutionary diagnostic and therapeutic concepts. And as they begin to heal they become your best advertisers.

PHONE CONSULTATIONS WITH DR. ROGERS

Many people are stuck. They have an undiagnosable condition. Or they have a label but have been unable to get well. Or they have a "dead-end" label which means nothing more can be done. And many are not able to find a physician who is trained in what our 9 books explore.

These people could benefit from a personal consultation with Dr. Sherry Rogers to explore what diagnostic and treatment options may exist that they or their physicians are not aware of. For this reason we offer prepaid, scheduled phone consultations with the doctor. These can be scheduled through the office by calling (315) 488-2856.

If you wish to send copies of your medical reports and/or also have your doctor on the line, this can be helpful as well. Reports must be received at least 3 weeks prior to the consult and not be on fax paper. They should be copies and not originals as they are not returnable. Do not send records without first having secured a scheduled appointment time, for records without an appointment are discarded.

Because you have not come to the office and been examined, you are not considered a patient (although you could elect to become one). In spite of that, you can learn what tests your physician could order and what plans you could follow. If he needs help in interpreting the tests, a scheduled follow-up consultation can allow you to explore treatment options with specific nutrient and other treatment suggestions. The point is, you do not have to be alone without guidance in your quest for wellness. And you owe it to yourself to explore the options that you might otherwise never even have heard of.

PRESTIGE PUBLISHING
P.O. BOX 3068
Syracuse, NY 13220
(800) 846-ONUS (6687) ◊ (315) 455-7862

HARD-COVER BOOKS

Depression Cured at Last!... $24.95

SOFT-COVER BOOKS

The E.I. Syndrome Revised... $17.95
You Are What You Ate.. $12.95
Tired or Toxic?... $17.95
Macro Mellow.. $12.95
The Cure Is In The Kitchen.. $14.95
Wellness Against All Odds... $17.95
Scientific Basis Environmental Medicine $17.95
Chemical Sensitivity.. $ 3.95

SPANISH TRANSLATIONS

Cansancio o Intoxicacion? $30.00
La Cura Se Encuentra En La Cocina............................. $30.00

Environmental Video 16 minute VHS........................... $12.95

TOTAL HEALTH: monthly newsletter on
current wellness and healing information/1 year $39.95
Mold Plates (one room).. $25.00
Formaldehyde Spot Test Kit $45.00
Slide show for physicians $333.00

Telephone consultations available with Dr. Rogers.
Contact Dr. Rogers' office (315) 488-2856 to schedule.

Shipping/Handling: Hard cover books $5.00 per single book/$2.00 each
additional book. All other books and products $4.00 per single item/$1.00
each additional item.

Name _____
Address _____
City _____ State_____ Zip _____
NYS residents add 7% sales tax.   Amount Enclosed $_____
❒ Check   ❒ Money Order   ❒ Visa/Mastercard
Card Number _____ Exp. _____
Signature _____